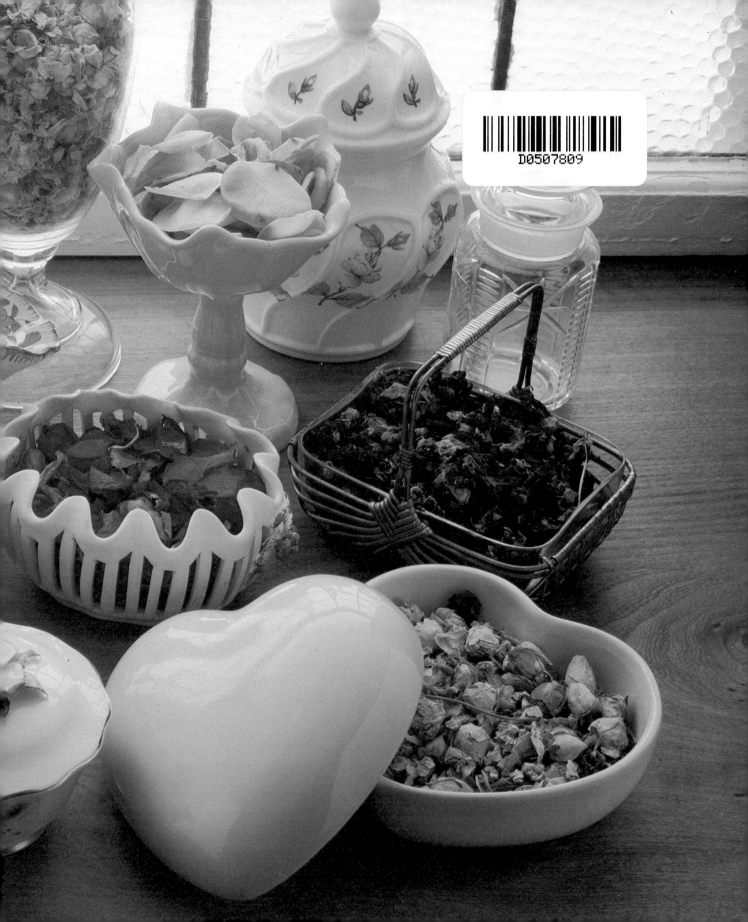

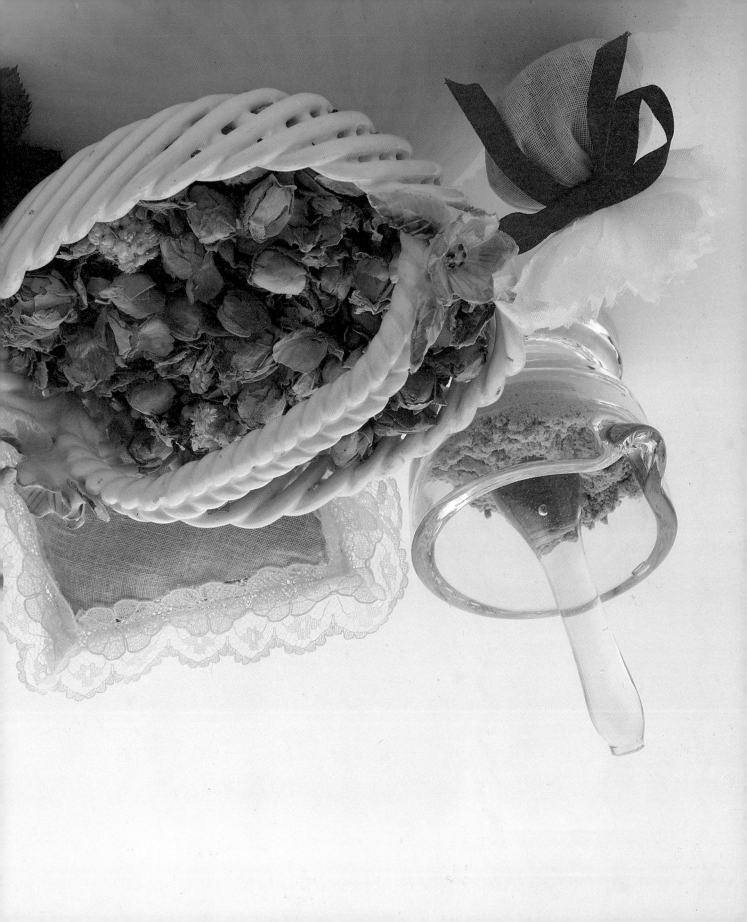

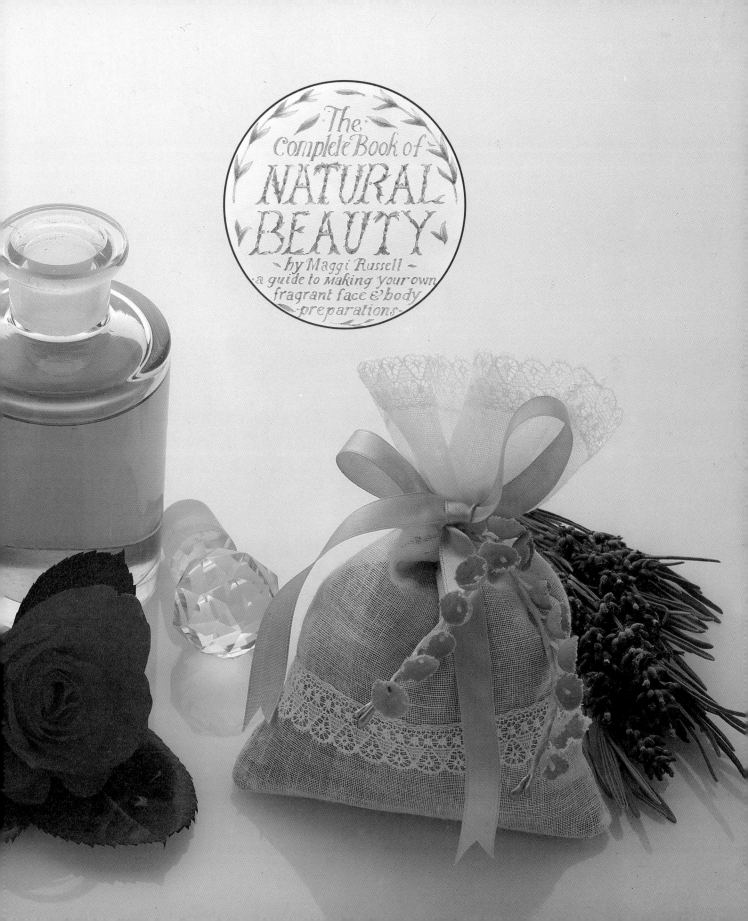

The
Complete Book of
NATURAL
BEAUTY

by Maggi Russell
a guide to making your own
fragrant face & body
preparations

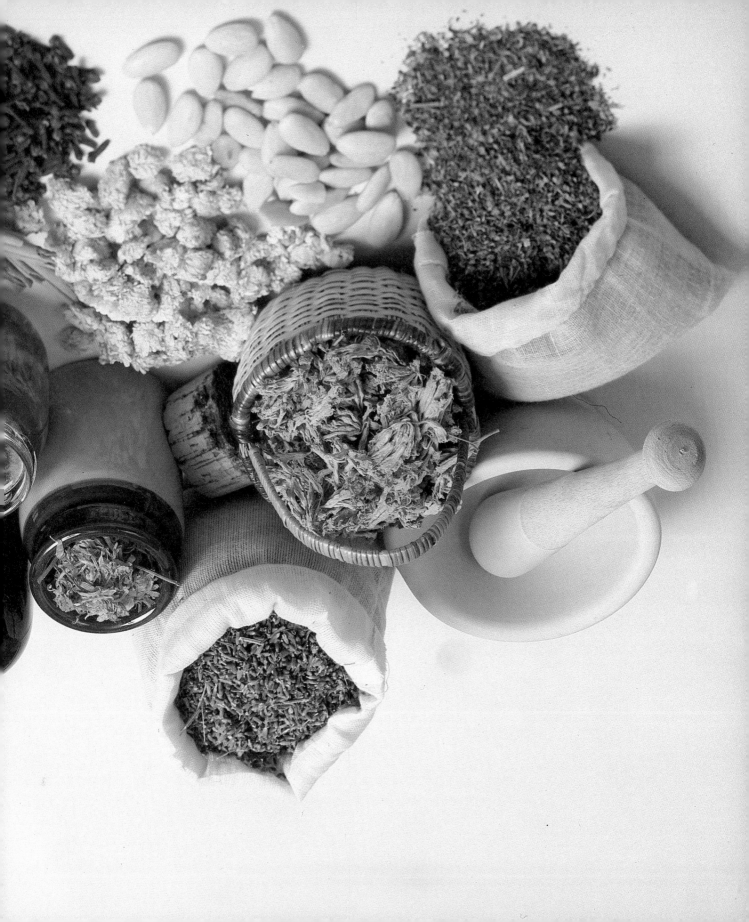

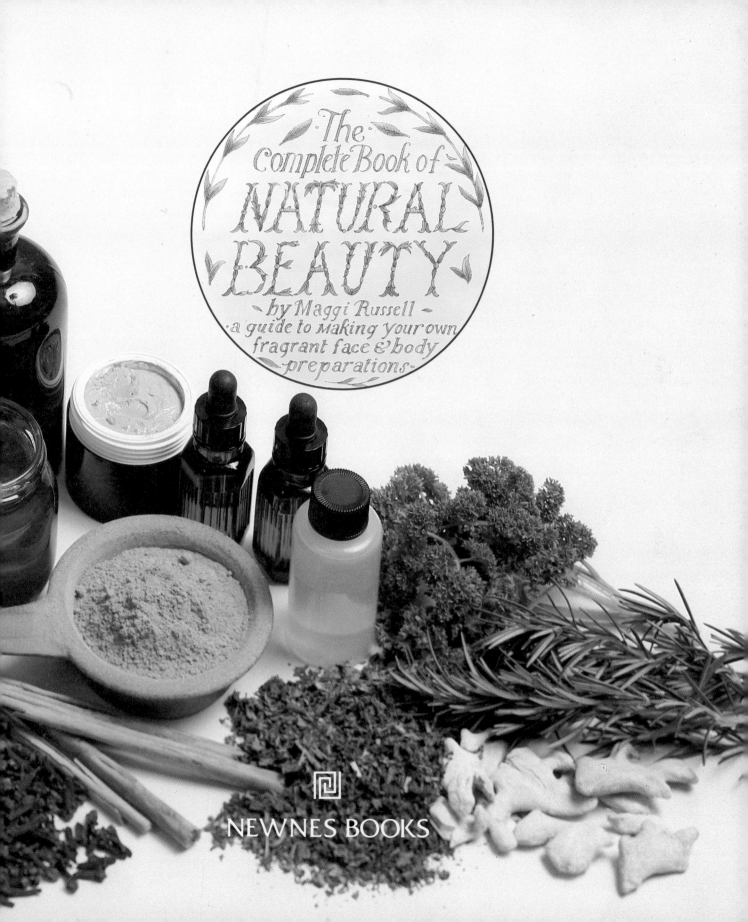

The Complete Book of NATURAL BEAUTY

- by Maggi Russell -
- a guide to making your own fragrant face & body preparations -

NEWNES BOOKS

Editor: Mary Lambert
Art editor: Caroline Dewing
Picture editor: Moira McIlroy
Black and white illustrations by Vana Haggerty
Cover and colour illustrations by Ian Beck

Published by Newnes Books, a division
of The Hamlyn Publishing Group Limited,
84-88, The Centre, Feltham, Middlesex, England
and distributed for them by
Hamlyn Distribution Services Limited,
Sanders Lodge Estate, Rushden, Northants, England

Any editorial queries should be addressed to
Marshall Cavendish Books Limited.

Any trade queries should be addressed to
Newnes Books.

ISBN   0 600 35897 6

Printed in Hong Kong

Contents

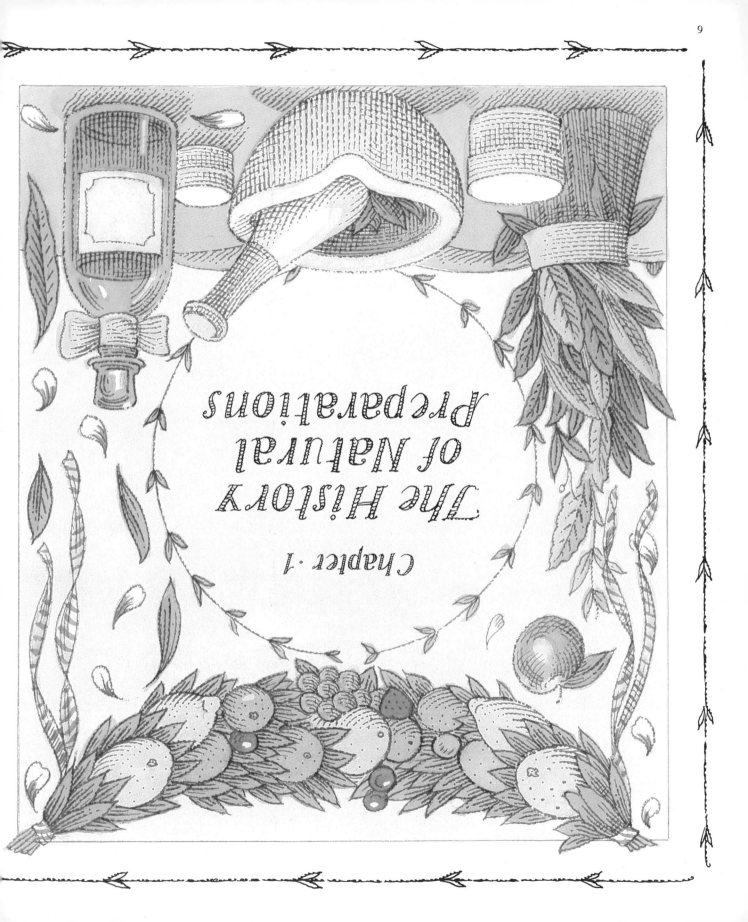

Chapter · 1

The History of Natural Preparations

Women have been preoccupied with trying to make themselves more beautiful for hundreds of years – it is certainly no recent phenomenon! The famous beauties of history have passed on their secrets in much the same way as film stars do today, – Cleopatra was just as fanatical about her baths of asses' milk as Jane Fonda is with her aerobics! Until the 19th century cosmetics were either homemade or concocted by physicians. Marie Antoinette, wife of Louis XVI, kept her oily skin under control with a cleansing milk of cream, lemon juice and brandy, while Lady Hamilton, Nelson's mistress, favoured a homemade strawberry astringent. Madame de Pompadour, extravagant mistress of Louis XV, kept her servants continuously on the run collecting armfuls of wild herbs for her aromatic baths, while Ann Boleyn, one of Henry VIII's wives, delighted in self-indulgence and often bathed in wine, which was then drunk by her courtiers with much ribaldry!

Commercial products

Today, we have a multi-million pound cosmetic industry offering face, body and hair preparations that promise to remove wrinkles, feed the skin, dissolve flab and thicken the hair. Many of them claim to be able to do this by adding 'herbal' ingredients to their products. A truly herbal product contains no chemicals and no preservatives, which means they do not last long and can only be made a few jars at a time. Commercial manufacturers have to make creams in batches of thousands, and give them an extended shelf-life of months or years by adding chemical preservatives. These products are designed to look extremely attractive, to feel and smell good and also to be beneficial to the skin, so artificial colourings, perfumes and pearlising agents are also added to make the cream or shampoo look more appealing. They are then tested (sometimes cruelly) on animals to make sure they will not irritate human skin. Packaging is of fundamental importance to catch the consumer's eye, and anything prettily bottled and labelled with pictures of flowers is bound to sell well. But with a little thought, a little research and experimentation, you can make your own cosmetics more cheaply than commercial products, and feel assured that the face cream you made, for example, is purer, fresher and more likely to do your skin good than anything you can buy in a shop. You can be in control of how much or how little of a chosen herb or organic ingredient to add to be sure of its beneficial action, and you do not need to add chemical preservatives as you are very likely to use up all of your homemade cosmetics long before they start deteriorating.

To make your own creams and lotions you can use the same recipes that our great-grandmothers used, which they in turn found in family recipe books passed down through the generations. But now you can adapt and refine them to make them smoother and easier to use by adding a little harmless technology.

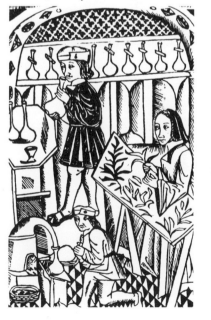

Since ancient times people have used herbs for their medicinal, cosmetic and fragrant properties. This sixteenth-century apothecary and his assistants are drying and preparing herbs for medicines and beauty aids which were then sold to the public.

The history of herbal cosmetics

How was it first discovered that plants could affect the condition of the skin? It most certainly happened by trial and error as prehistoric people discovered that the sticky gum from trees could help to heal hunting wounds, and certain leaves used as bandages had a cooling and soothing effect. The ancient Egyptians are believed to have been the first people to prepare scented oils for bathing, massaging and embalming. The Egyptian women also discovered the benefits of using honey masks to improve the complexion thousands of years before the birth of Christ. The ancient Chinese soon discovered the benefits of natural ingredients and wrote down many hundreds of recipes for herbal ointments and poultices. Galen, the Greek physician concocted the first face cream 1,700 years ago, using white wax, spermaceti, almond oil, rosewater and borax. His cream recipe has become the basis for many face creams that are made today.

How plants were judged

Today the science of pharmacology studies exactly how and why the chemical constituents of plants have a medicinal action on the human body. This is a far cry from the days when herbal magicians gathered their plants in the wild and designated them for a particular medical task by using a theory called the 'Doctrine of Signatures'. In this way the potential healing power of a plant was judged by its outward appearance and some fancied resemblance to a particular part of the human anatomy. So kidney vetch was named and used to help treat kidney complaints because its leaves resembled this organ in shape. The colour of a plant, too, was believed to correspond to a bodily condition – red flowers were thought to purify the blood, yellow flowers to lighten the hair and so forth. Sometimes these ancient herbalists were uncannily accurate, sometimes not, but they were the pioneers of the systematic, scientific study of botany which has over the years discovered countless herbs with medicinal or skin-refining properties.

The active properties of plants

Today these herbal properties have been recognized as dividing into certain active constituents. These consist of carbohydrates, amino acids, volatile oils, glycosides, terpenoids and alkaloids. There are many other complex compounds whose chemical natures are as yet unknown. In simplified terms, these active constituents act on the exterior of the body as antiseptics, astringents, lighteners, lubricators and softeners. The essential oils of plants are highly aromatic, producing fragrant smells that are inhaled and consequently act on the nervous system producing soothing or stimulating effects. They also contain azulene which lightens the skin, and antiseptics which promote the healing of skin disorders.

The tannins, mucilage and vitamins in plants cleanse, nourish and tighten the skin, and substances like allantoin from the comfrey herb have

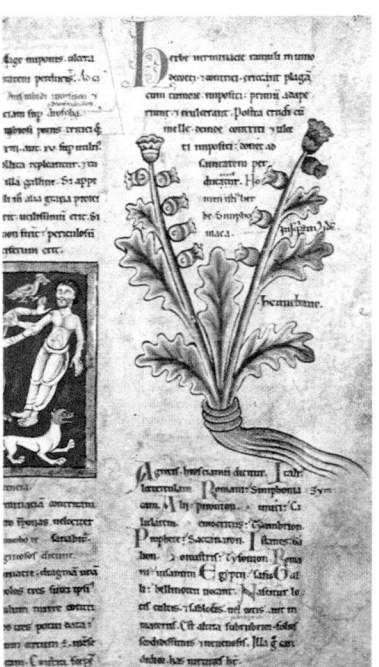

In the past the possible healing powers of a plant were gauged by its colour, what it looked like and whether it resembled a particular part of the body. This thirteenth-century manuscript depicts a man suffering from the bite of a mad dog, and on the right, henbane is illustrated, the plant used to try and cure him.

remarkable skin restoring properties. The basis for all this knowledge we have acquired today comes from the writings and practice of the herbalists.

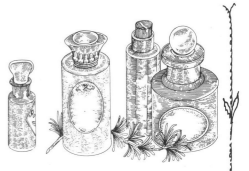

Cosmetics today

Skin and hair preparations which were based on ancient herbal knowledge remained much the same until the late 19th century, when Helena Rubenstein's mother discovered a Hungarian chemist making a face cream from a mixture of herbs, essence of almonds and bark of an evergreen tree. As she grew up, Helena Rubenstein started to use this cream. She was so impressed with its qualities that she began producing it with the cooperation of the chemist. It became the first product, therefore, of her now international cosmetic industry. She was also one of the first people to take a scientific approach to skincare.

As more experimentation was undertaken with making synthetic cosmetics, they soon became extremely popular and the ancient herbal approach was forgotten. Earlier this century, scientific interest in natural substances was virtually non-existent and synthetics were thought to be the answer to everything. The mystique surrounding the use of herbs was found too woolly for the technological age. Thankfully, today, this view has changed and natural products have become popular and again modern technology is now being used to investigate the natural properties of herbs under strictly scientific conditions.

Homemade cosmetics

Why bother to make your own cosmetics? Because not only is it great fun, highly creative and reasonably cheap, but because you can make the perfect creams and lotions for your own individual needs, knowing that all the ingredients are pure, fresh and full of properties that will help your skin.

You can grow or gather many useful herbs and flowers for cosmetic recipes, or alternatively you can buy a wide selection, ready-dried, from herbalists. It is important to try and obtain them from a reputable source rather than buying the bottled varieties found in grocery stores, as herbalists prepare and dry their herbs carefully to retain their active properties. Organic ingredients such as fruits, grains, honey and eggs are easily obtainable from shops and supermarkets, and all the other ingredients, such as waxes, oils and natural preservatives can be bought or ordered through any major chemist.

When you have made your cosmetics, you can keep them in pretty bottles and pots with decorative labels so that they make perfect presents to outclass many a shop-bought product. They are less likely to cause allergic reactions than commercial, preservative-filled cosmetics, and you can adapt and experiment with the ingredients and perfumes in the recipes to suit yourself. Once you have achieved the right blend in your products, you may never want to buy a commercial cosmetic again!

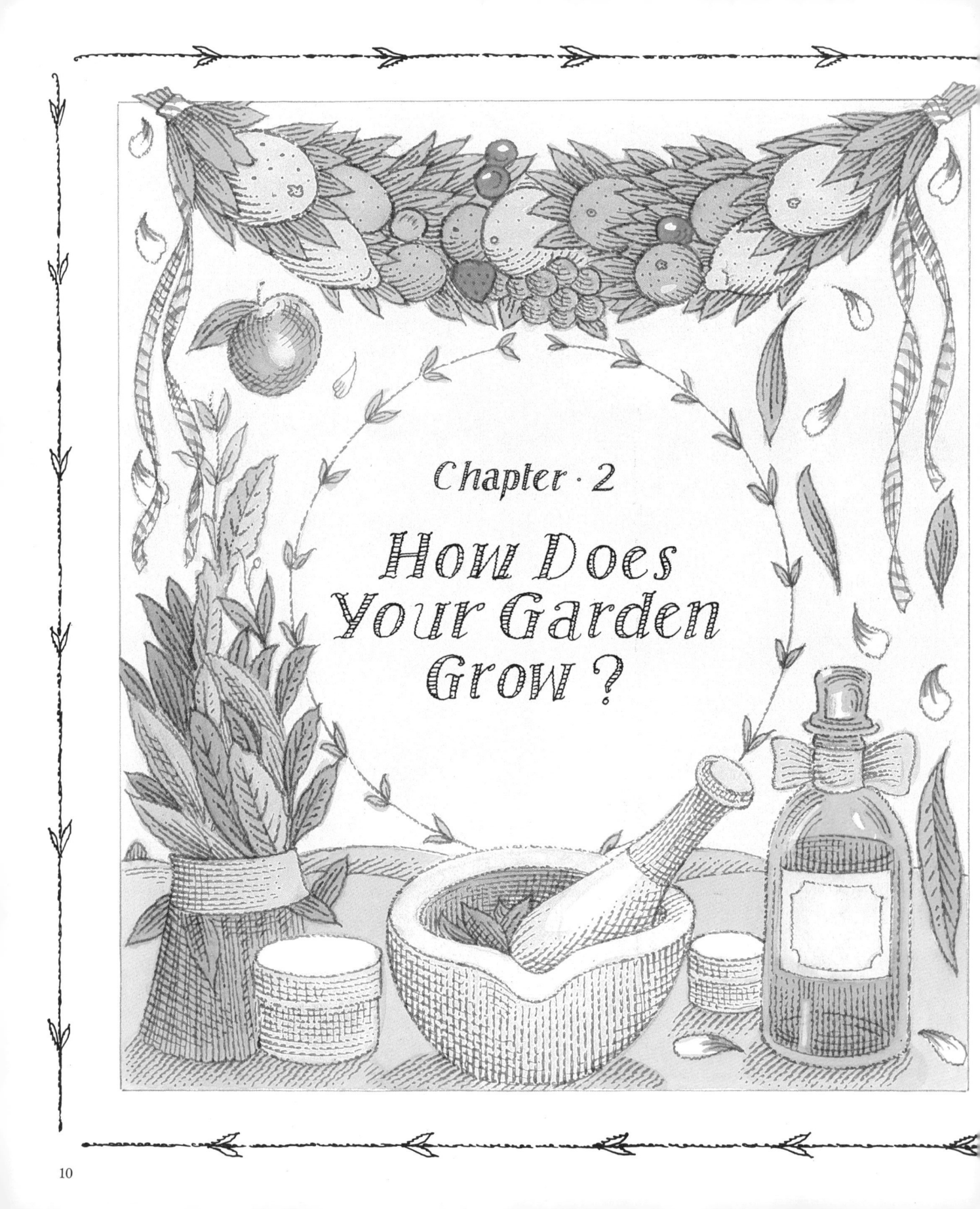

Chapter · 2

How Does Your Garden Grow ?

In ancient times people had little need for herb gardens – all the plants they wanted for their medicinal or culinary purposes grew plentifully in fields and woods. But by the Middle Ages monasteries were cultivating their own large gardens in which they grew a wide variety of herbs, and grand houses soon started to do the same. Private gardens were planted with suitable herbs to cure the family ills, and scented flowers to make sweet waters. The mistress of the house would oversee the distillation of perfumes in her still room, and servants were employed for the sole purpose of tending and gathering the herbs. By Elizabethan times the herb garden was as important to the house as the kitchen, as herbs were used for countless domestic functions, not least of which as air fresheners to fumigate the rooms with pleasant smells.

As a bonus to all their practical uses, herbs are an attractive and fragrant addition to any garden. If you already possess a well-cultivated plot, you are sure to have many useful herbs and flowers at your disposal. Or you can add to those you have already to create a well-balanced selection. But even if all you own is a tiny garden, a few metres square, with a couple of neglected flowerbeds, you can still transform this into a delightful, fragrant and useful herb garden.

The lack of any garden at all should not deter you from growing the smaller plants – even a tiny patio, window boxes or indoor areas can produce a healthy crop. Growing your own herbs is much more fulfilling than buying the dried variety in packets, and you will always have fresh herbs at your disposal. But for those without 'green fingers', dried herbs will be perfectly adequate and produce cosmetics that are just as beneficial.

Before deciding which ones to grow, look through the recipes to see which herbs most suit your beauty needs, and check the *Growing Guide For Garden Herbs And Flowers* on pages 36-37 to see which are most likely to thrive in the growing conditions you have to offer. Herbs that can still be found growing plentifully in the wild are not really worth growing as they can take over the garden, but some like nettles, camomile and yarrow are very beneficial to the soil, and actually help to nurse other herbs growing near them.

Herbs are generally very hardy and minimal tending is needed, but it is important that they are grown in the right position. Most herbs like plenty of sunshine but some types prefer shade, and some are more prone to the ravages of insects and disease others. The following guidelines will set you on your way to growing your first herbs, but to help you become an expert gardener it is recommended that you invest in a good gardening book.

Growing herbs in one flowerbed

If you are restricted to just one flowerbed, a small plot 3.6m (4yd) by 1.8m (2 yd), would be large enough to supply herbs for most of your needs. When you plant your herbs make sure you balance the plot by placing the tall ones at the back and the small ones at the front.

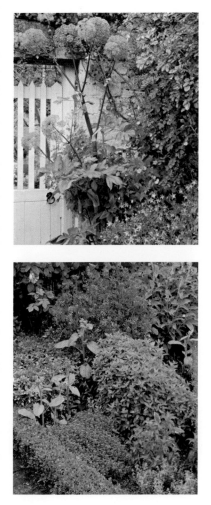

Below: Most herbs are very hardy and require little care, so if they are not cut back they will spread rapidly to give a wild, natural looking garden.

Bottom: A more formal, ordered effect can be achieved by planting your herbs in neat rows, with the tallest ones at the back and the bushiest ones clipped to form dividing hedges.

The right soil

Most herbs came originally from hot, dry climates so they do not need a rich soil, and a light, sandy or peaty one is best. Covering the soil with a 2.5cm (1in) layer of peat helps to keep it from drying out or cracking up in the cold weather. Put the peat down during the spring and dampen it first before spreading. Do not use proprietary fertilizers – soil conditions closest to the herbs' natural habitat in the wild are best. You can, however, make your own organic fertilizer by starting a compost heap with fallen leaves, vegetable peelings, lawn mowings and food remains. A strong infusion of nettles also makes a good fertilizer as well as a natural insect repellent. Do not use chemical pesticides as these will taint the herbs. More important than feeding herbs is providing good drainage so that the roots do not become waterlogged. A heavy soil can be made more crumbly by adding some drainage material such as a light friable loam. Ask for a suitable mixture at a gardening centre.

Growing from seedlings

Potted seedlings from a nursery are the best buy when starting a herb garden. Make the transition from pot to flowerbed gradually, by leaving the plants outside in their pots to become acclimatized to the cooler weather conditions. Remove the seedling by inverting and squeezing the base of the plastic pot, so that the rootlets and surrounding soil come out in one piece. Plant the herb and its soil into the earth with the rootlets 2.5cm (1in) beneath the surface and water.

Growing from seeds

Seeds in packets are sold with detailed growing instructions. Most need planting in the spring, after the risk of frosts has passed. Mixing the seeds with a little sand helps them to retain moisture and deters slugs. Water well after planting. When the seedlings have grown 5cm (2in) and have four leaves, thin them out to give each growing plant more room.

Lawn herbs

Some herbs that are thought of as weeds grow profusely amongst the grass on the lawn. Clover, yarrow and camomile are the most common ones. As well as being useful to you they act as fertilizers for the grass, so it makes sense to let them merge in.

Indoor growing

Herbs can be grown indoors or on patios in large tubs or terracotta pots, but old sinks and tin baths will do just as well. Do not cram them into small pots as the larger ones provide similar growing conditions to outside and the soil will stay moist longer and be more nutritious. Containers must have holes underneath to allow excess water to drain out, otherwise the roots will

A small patio can be transformed into a fragrant garden by planting herbs in large containers. Old sinks and chimney pots make practical and attractive containers, but if using metal or wooden tubs make sure to treat them first with paint or preservative to stop rust and mould developing.

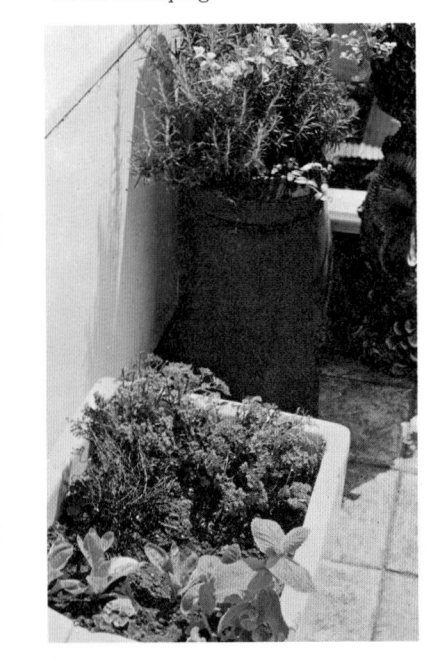

become waterlogged and start to rot. If they are made of tin or metal they should be treated first with two coats of paint to stop rust and mould, and wooden ones will need treating inside with a wood preservative that is not harmful to plants.

Compost and watering

You should not use earth dug up from the garden as it will become waterlogged and encourages fungi. Use a well-balanced compost such as John Innes Number 2 or 3. This is sterilized and is nutritious, as well as being light and porous; add charcoal granules to keep the compost sweet. The roots must be able to feed, but moisture must be able to drain away. Never over-water your herbs – pour water into the trays on which the pots stand, and throw away any surplus water after two hours. Only water the top soil if it appears dry.

The right position

Keep sun-loving plants on the window ledge or sill, and shade-loving plants away from direct sunlight. Avoid placing them in draughts, but make sure the rooms are well ventilated. If you have centrally-heated rooms attach humidifiers to each radiator to keep some moisture in the air. Turn plants occasionally as they always grow towards the light. When taking leaves and sprigs for use, take them from all around the plant so that its growth does not become unbalanced.

Window boxes

If your window boxes are made of wood, treat them with a non-toxic wood

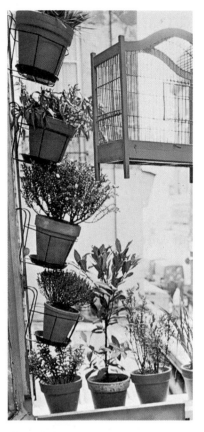

Above: The smaller herbs grow well in terracotta pots, but should be turned regularly as they grow towards the light. Keep them on small trays and water the trays rather than the top soil, so that the roots can take as much moisture as they need.

Left: Basil grows well in small containers. Taking sprigs from the top will help the plant to thicken up and stop it becoming too straggly.

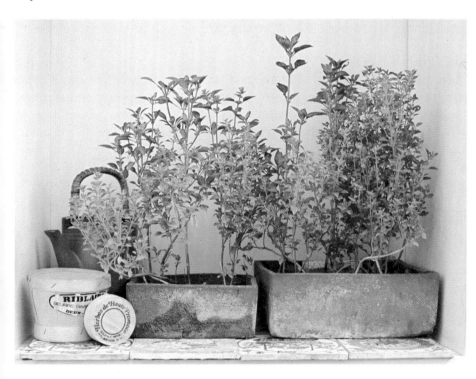

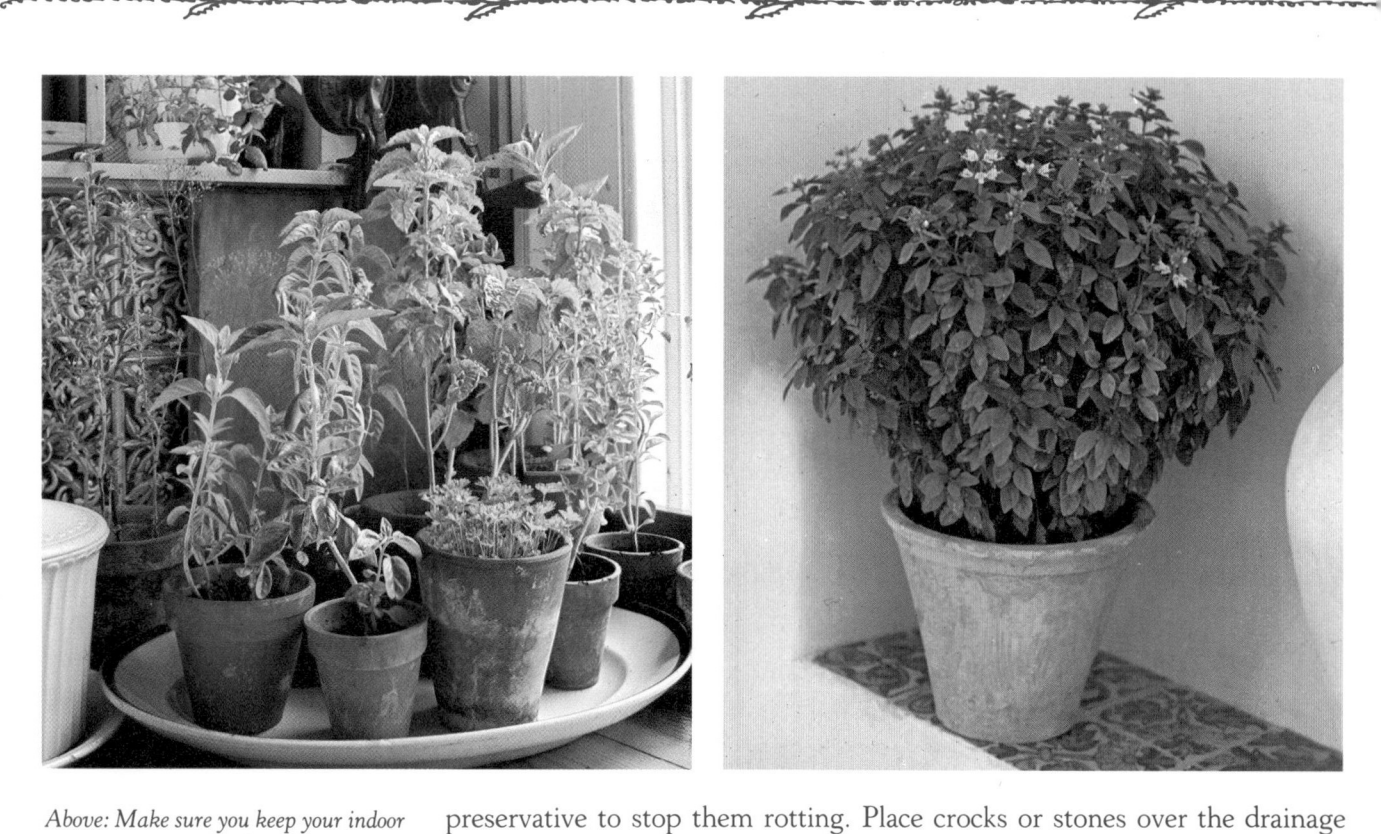

Above: Make sure you keep your indoor herbs in the right position. Some such as balm, parsley, thyme and fennel like plenty of sunlight and grow well on window sills.

Above right: Some herbs such as mint prefer a shady position and grow very well in a corner away from the window. Taking sprigs from the top help it to grow into a bushy, attractive houseplant.

preservative to stop them rotting. Place crocks or stones over the drainage holes and again use a well-balanced compost with added charcoal granules. Water from above when the compost feels slightly dry. Herbs like balm, parsley, sage and thyme are ideal for window boxes. Plant in the spring.

Hanging baskets
Metal hanging baskets will last longer if you paint them before use, plastic ones need no preparation. Line all baskets with sphagnum moss from garden shops to absorb moisture and keep the soil in place. Use a well-balanced soil and charcoal granules. Allow the soil to settle for a few days, then plant the taller herbs in the centre and the smaller, trailing ones on the outside. Water by leaving to soak in a bucket of water three times a week in summer and as required in winter, and spray frequently all over.

Herbs in the wild
Sadly many herbs no longer grow as profusely in the wild as they used to, because of modern pollution and chemical pesticides. But if you live in the country you can still find plenty of useful plants growing in fields and woods. Invest in a gardening book which has colour photographs or illustrations so that you can readily identify them. You should be able to find camomile, dandelion, comfrey, marshmallow, mullein, soapwort, valerian, pine and lime in plenty. Never take the whole plant, just a few sprigs.

Do not pick herbs growing by roadsides or those that grow near large

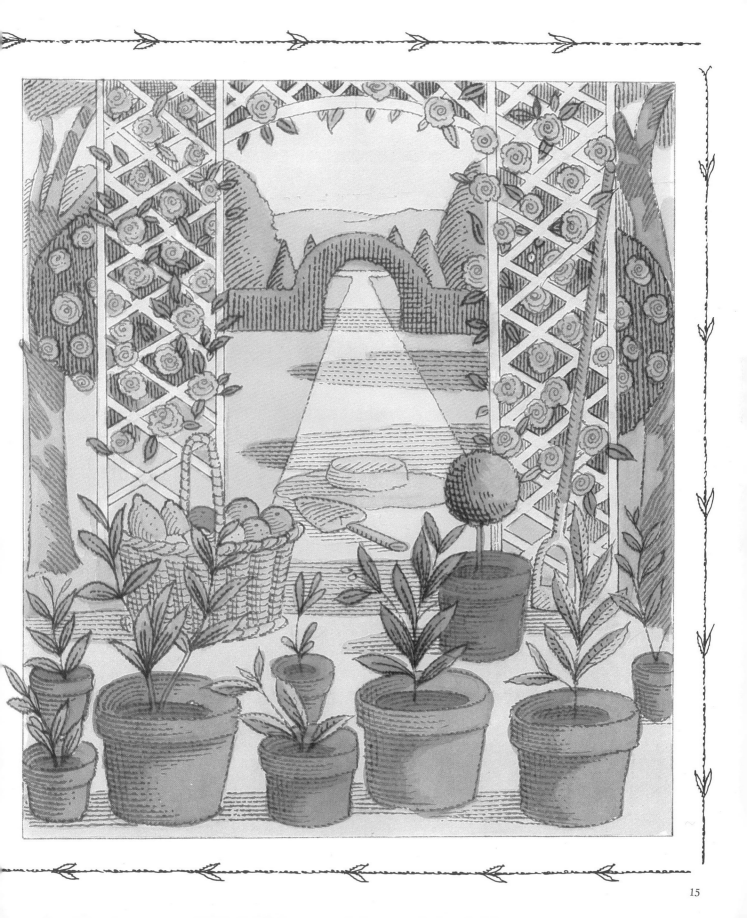

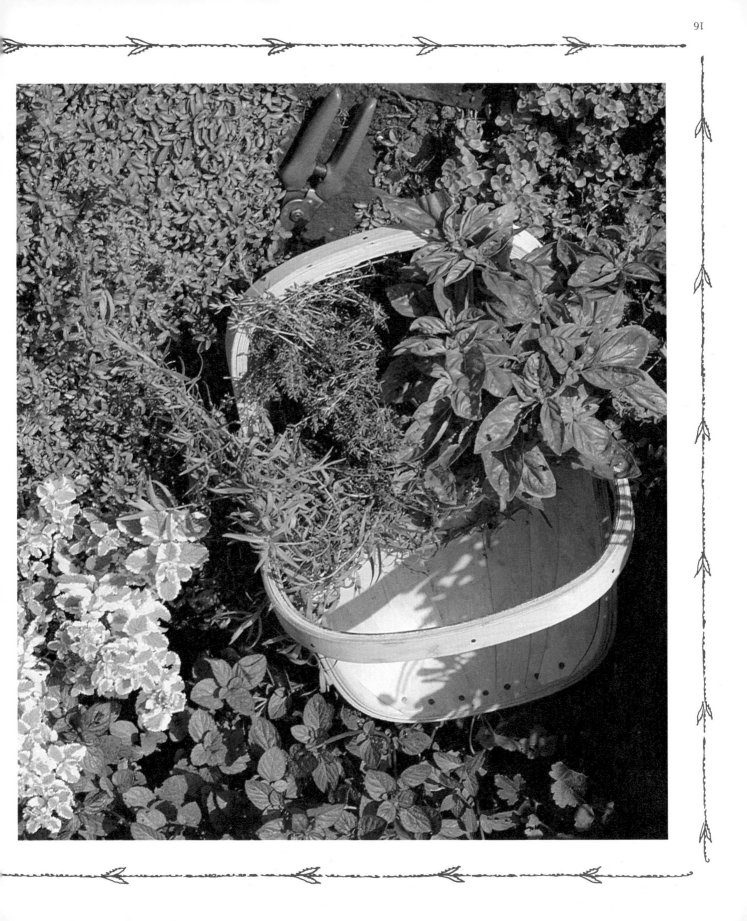

cultivated fields, as they are likely to be contaminated by carbon monoxide fumes and the chemical fertilizers used by farmers. Never pick herbs that are yellow, faded, wilted or insect-eaten as they will be past their best. If in doubt of the identity of a plant do not pick it. Foxglove leaves are poisonous but look remarkably like comfrey, while hemlock can be mistaken for parsley.

Gathering herbs, flowers and fruits

Herb gathering is a meticulous art. Plants should be harvested when young, fully grown and healthy, at exactly the right moment when their therapeutic qualities are at a peak. This is known as the 'balsamic moment', when the plant is producing its most active ingredients. This moment comes during the late spring or summer, in the early morning on a dry day, after the dew has evaporated, or in the late afternoon. Wet flowers are prone to mildew once picked. Taking flowers and sprigs from the top of the plant will help it to produce more shoots.

Herbage (leaves, stalks and flowers together) should be collected just as the plant begins to flower.

Leaves should be picked young, but fully grown, before the plant flowers.

Flowers can be collected at the start of the plant's flowering season. Try to pick them just as they open up and before they have been pollinated. Flowers continue to open after they have been separated from the plant.

Fruits should be collected as they begin to ripen – not while they are still green but just before they would be ready to eat.

Seeds are removed from mature fruits. If seeds are exposed on stems take the whole stem indoors and hang it upside down over a tray then wait for the seeds to fall.

Berries should be picked when ripe but not soft.

Bark should be cut in spring when the flow of sap is at its maximum. Use a knife with care – do not just strip it off as you are likely to take too much and damage the tree. Only cut from the larger branches.

Roots are dug up in the autumn when the plant is preparing for winter, or in the spring. Lift the plant gently and shake the roots free of soil. Wash them under a tap and dry thoroughly with a towel.

Equipment for collection of herbs

Garden scissors are useful to cut stems of plants, or use secateurs for the woodier varieties. Flowers and leaves can be picked with your fingers. Handle all plants very gently so as not to bruise or crush them, and place them in a large flat basket or a tray, separating each type into small piles. Do not use plastic bags to collect herbs as they will trap heat and moisture and encourage the plants to rot.

Take your herb collection indoors, and sort and separate them ready for the drying process.

It is very important to pick your herbs at the right time and in the right way. Flowers should be picked just as they open at the start of the flowering season, and be handled very gently so they are not bruised. A flat basket is ideal for carrying your herb collection home, as you can store each type in separate piles.

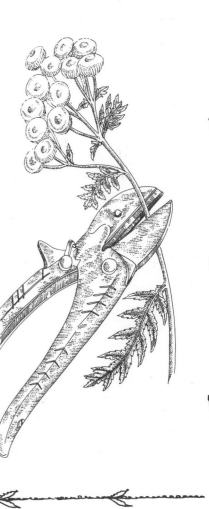

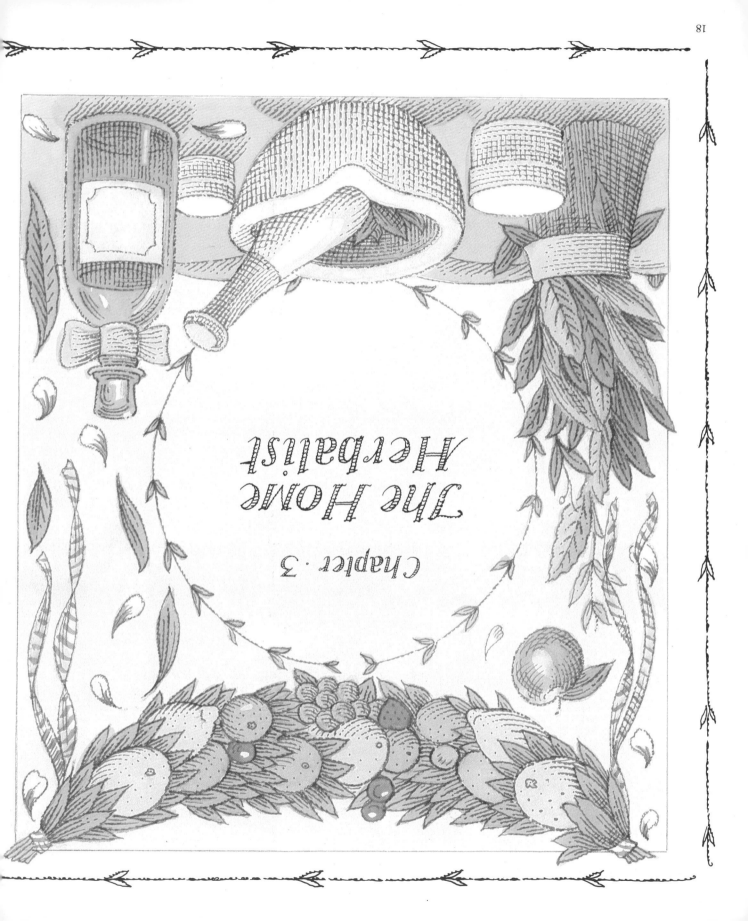

Chapter · 3

The HOME
Herbalist

Ideally herbs should be used fresh, but this is not always possible, especially in winter months. The next best options are to dry or freeze the herbs you have gathered in the summer.

To freeze herbs simply make sure they are free from dirt and moisture before cutting them into small twigs. To store them use wax cartons like the ones sold with yoghurt, or alternatively plastic cartons. Label them clearly, then defrost in the cartons before use.

Drying leaves, flowers and stems

To dry herbs means to remove their water content, and if it is done quickly and efficiently most of the active constituents and fragrances of the herbs should stay intact. The best method is to hang the complete stems in small bunches in a warm, dark dry place – an airing cupboard is ideal. Do not crowd them all together as it is important to let air circulate around them. Hang them in your kitchen, if it is dry and warm, but keep them away from cooking as the steam will impede the drying process. Do not hang in a garage if you keep a car in there because of the carbon monoxide fumes.

If you have not got room to hang herbs, you can make trays for them. Cover wooden frames with nylon netting or cheesecloth, cover with herbs, then stack the trays so that the air can circulate freely between each layer. If making trays sounds too much like hard work, spread your herbs on clean dry paper, and turn them frequently, particularly in the first 24 hours. The herbs are dry once they feel crisp and crackly to the touch. Flowers will look papery and the leaves will look parched. If you are only going to be using the flowers or leaves from a herb, remove them from the twigs for storing. The dried twigs can be added to open fires for a delightful aroma.

Drying roots and seeds

First trim away all the fibrous parts clinging to the roots, then scrub them with clean water and pat dry with kitchen paper. Leave them to dry for an hour in a warm room. Then cut into 1.5cm (½in) lengths and spread out on drying trays or paper. Once they break when bent they are thoroughly dry. If they are still leathery they need further drying.

Seeds are dry once they crack between your fingernails. Stir them regularly to turn them.

Storing

Store each variety of herb separately in green or amber glass jars with well fitting stoppers. It is important to keep herbs away from sunlight to preserve their active principles. Also keep the jars away from damp and heat and do not store herbs in tins as these can affect the flavour. Label and date each jar, and use up the contents as quickly as possible, they will not be useful after a year, although roots last longer. Store the jars in a dark cupboard.

If you see beads of moisture forming in the jar after the first few days, it

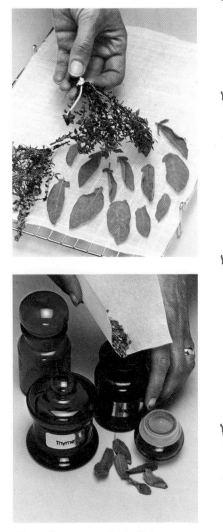

Above: Store your dried herbs in opaque glass bottles and keep these tightly closed. The bottles should then be stored in a cupboard away from the light.

Top: Dry your herbs by spreading them on wooden or metal drying racks. Large leaves should be dried separately while sprigs with small leaves can be tied in loose bundles.

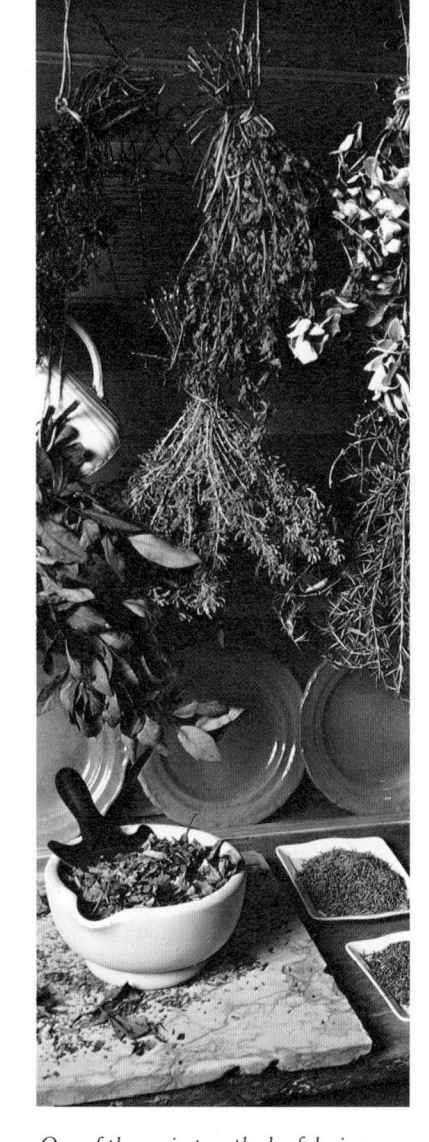

One of the easiest methods of drying herbs is to hang them upside-down in bunches in a warm, dry place. If hanging in the kitchen keep away from water vapour caused by cooking as this will inhibit the drying process.

simply means the herb needs further drying. Empty out the contents and dry them again, then re-store in a dry bottle.

Preparing herbs for use

To release the vital properties contained in herbs, they need to be heated in water or steeped in oil, vinegar or alcohol. These methods make infusions, decoctions and macerations. From these basic techniques you can make all the herbal waters, oils, essences and extracts you need for cosmetic use.

Infusions

A tisane or herbal tea is simply a weak infusion, prepared by pouring boiling water over the herb, just like making a pot of Indian tea. Herbal tea mixtures are sold ready-prepared and are drunk hot and sweetened with honey. For cosmetic purposes, infusions of herbs need to be stronger than teas, but are prepared in exactly the same way.

To make a herbal infusion take 25g (1oz) of the dried herb or one and a half handfuls of the fresh one. Place it in a glass, china, pottery or enamel container – do not use plastic or metal which can destroy the delicate flavour of the herb. Use the purest water possible, a mild mineral water or purified water from the chemist. The heavy limestone content in tap water makes it too hard for the best results. Rainwater is also excellent.

Pour 600ml (1pt) of boiling water over the herb and cover the container tightly. Much of a herb's value is in its volatile oil which can evaporate when left open to the air. Allow the infusion to steep for at least 30 minutes. Strain through a plastic strainer or coffee filter paper before use. To double the strength of the infusion simply double the quantity of herb used.

An infusion can be stored in the fridge for up to three days – after that it may start fermenting and will have to be thrown away.

Decoctions

The tougher parts of a plant such as the roots, stalks, seeds and bark need more vigorous processing to give up their therapeutic qualities, so they have to be boiled *in* water. This method is called decoction.

Take 25g (1oz) of the dried or fresh root, bark, stalk or seeds and place in an enamel-coated or glass saucepan. Pour 600ml (1pt) of purified water over the herb and bring to the boil, then turn the heat down and simmer for 30 minutes. The liquid should be reduced to about half the quantity, but if it is boiling away too quickly, add more water. Strain through a plastic strainer or coffee filter paper into a glass or china container. Seal tightly and use as soon as possible. To make a double strength decoction simply double the amount of herb used. Wash utensils well after use.

Macerations

To macerate a herb means to steep it in oil, wine, vinegar or alcohol for anything from a few hours to several weeks. This method is used when the vital properties of the herb could be adversely affected by heat, or to make a preparation that will keep longer.

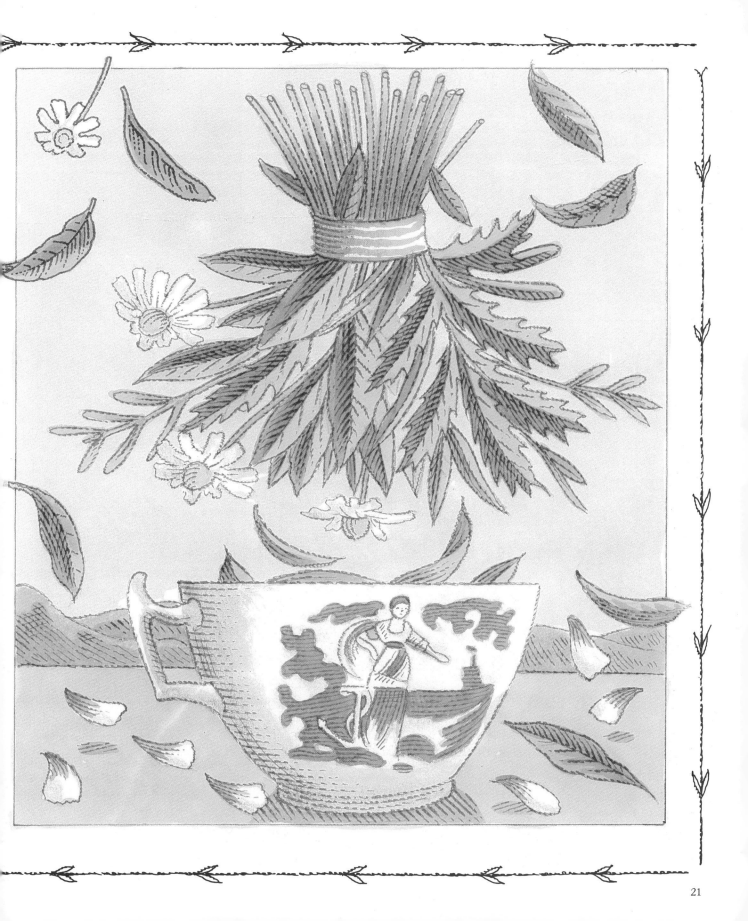

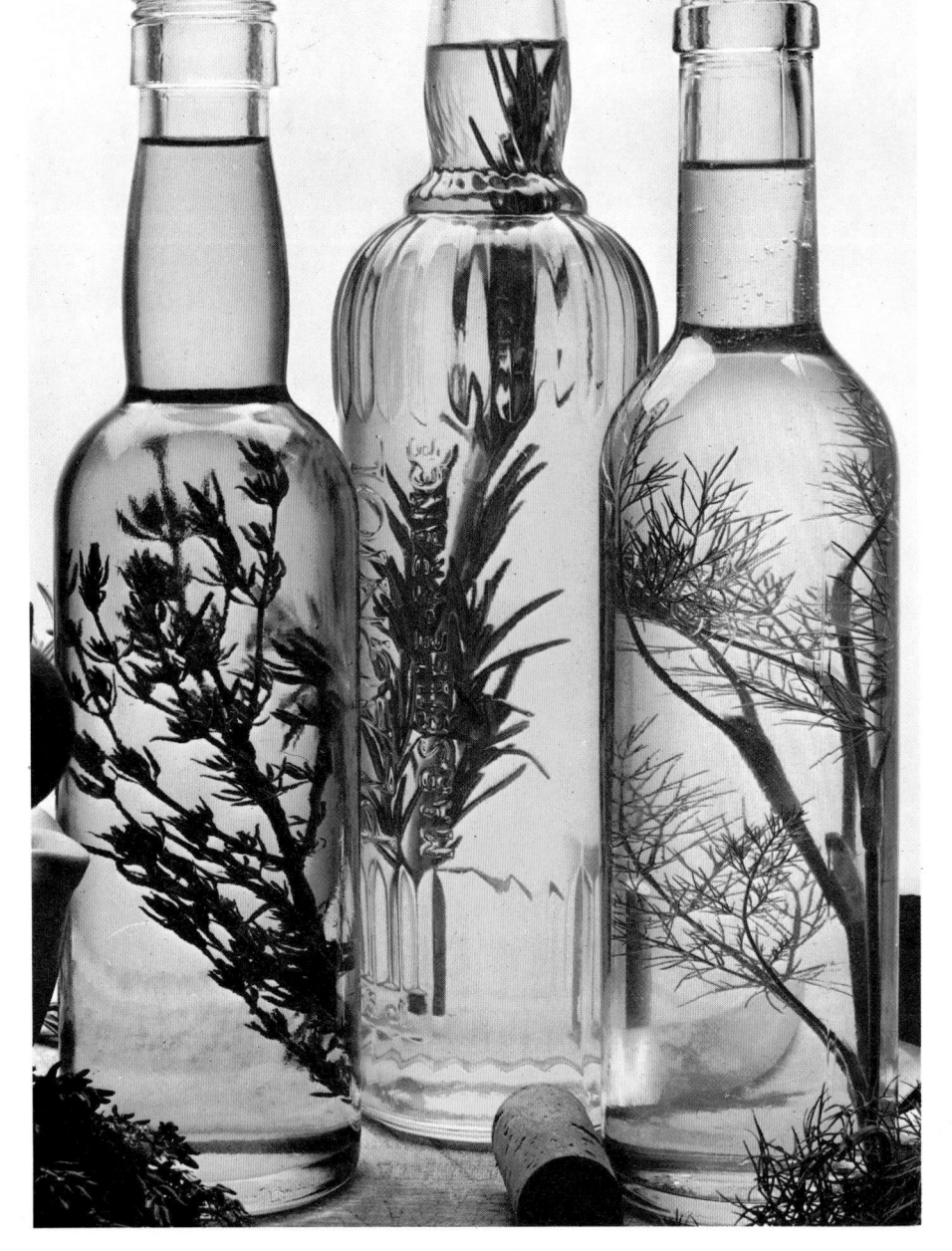

Herbal vinegars make wonderful facial astringents and hair rinses. They are easily made by adding sprigs of your chosen herb to cider or white wine vinegar and macerating for a short time. They can be left in the bottle while the vinegar is in use.

Herb oils Macerating in oil makes herb oils – do not confuse these with essential oils which are the actual unadulterated volatile oils of the herb itself. These cannot be extracted in any quantity without complicated equipment and techniques. But a herb or flower oil made by steeping the plant in a fine oil such as almond oil gives a fragrant oil ready for use alone or added to other ingredients.

Take 25g (1oz) of the dried herb or one and a half handfuls of the fresh herb, and pound with a pestle in a mortar to make a mulch. Empty the dried herb or the green mulch into a large screw-top jar and add a tablespoon of white wine, cider vinegar or vodka. Cover with a 600ml (1pt) of any vegetable oil such as sunflower, safflower, or olive oil, or for the finest results use sweet almond oil from the chemist's. To make less of the herb oil, simply halve these quantities. Screw the lid on tightly, after making sure that the jar is not too full so there is room to shake the contents vigorously.

It is important to keep the maceration warm for the herb's qualities to be extracted. In summer, place the jar in a sunny spot on a window sill, and shake every day for a month. In winter, place the jar on or above a radiator. When the time is up, try a little of the oil on your wrist to see if it smells strongly enough of the herb. If not, add this oil to another batch of herbs and repeat again. When the oil smells 'herby' enough, strain it through a nylon sieve to remove all the bits of the herb, mashing the herb into the sieve to extract every last drop of its qualities. Re-bottle in a clean, dark glass jar, seal tightly and store in a cool, dark place. Do not forget to label it with the name of the herb used, and the date.

Floral oils To make floral oils from dried flowerheads use the above technique, but when using fresh flowers the oil needs to be warmed to extract the fragrance, Highly scented flowers such as rose, jasmine, geranium, lilac, lavender and lily of the valley make excellent floral oils.

Pour 300ml (½pt) of sweet almond oil into the top pan of an enamel-coated double boiler, or into a small heat resistant bowl inside a larger saucepan. Fill the larger pan with enough water to stop the oil burning when the water is heated. Heat the larger pan until the oil is warm, then fill the oil with as many flowerheads as possible, cover the inner pot and leave on a very low heat to warm gently for two hours. Then squeeze all the oil from the flowers, remove them and replace with a fresh supply. Repeat the process every two hours until the perfume is strong when tested on your wrist. Do not forget to top up the water in the larger pan if some has evaporated. When the oil is strong enough, increase the heat and allow the oil to simmer until the flowers have dried up. Then strain through a plastic sieve into a dark glass bottle. Add one teaspoon of tincture of benzoin as a preservative, then seal, shake well, label and store in a cool dark place.

Herbal and flower essences and waters Essences are made by mixing two tablespoons of the herb or floral oil with 600ml (1pt) of cider or wine vinegar. To make less, just halve the quantities. Essences in turn can be used in making herbal and floral waters. Simply add a tablespoon of the essence to 600ml (1pt) of purified water, seal the bottle and shake well.

Herbal vinegars These are made by macerating the herb in vinegar instead of oil, and are ready after three days only. Use the same ratio of herbs – 25g (1oz) of the dried herb or one and a half handfuls of the fresh herb and 600ml (1pt) of cider or white wine vinegar. (Do not use malt vinegar, it is far too strong.) Use them as astringents and hair rinses.

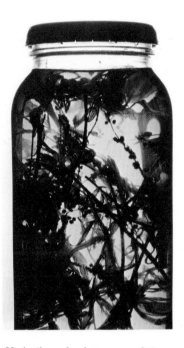

Herb oils are lovely to use on their own after a bath or when added to face and body lotions. They are made by macerating the herb in the oil for several weeks, then straining the mixture through a sieve.

Directory of ingredients to grow or buy

The following alphabetical listings include all the herbs, flowers, fruits, vegetables, oils and other miscellaneous ingredients you will need to prepare and make your own cosmetics. You may not need them all, so check the recipes first to see which ones you need to use, then look up the ingredient in one of the A-Z listings here to see how to grow it or obtain it.

An A to Z of herbs and flowers

All the herbs and flowers listed here have been valued since ancient times for their therapeutic and beauty-enhancing principles. They are all included in the recipes, some of which were made by women thousands of years ago.

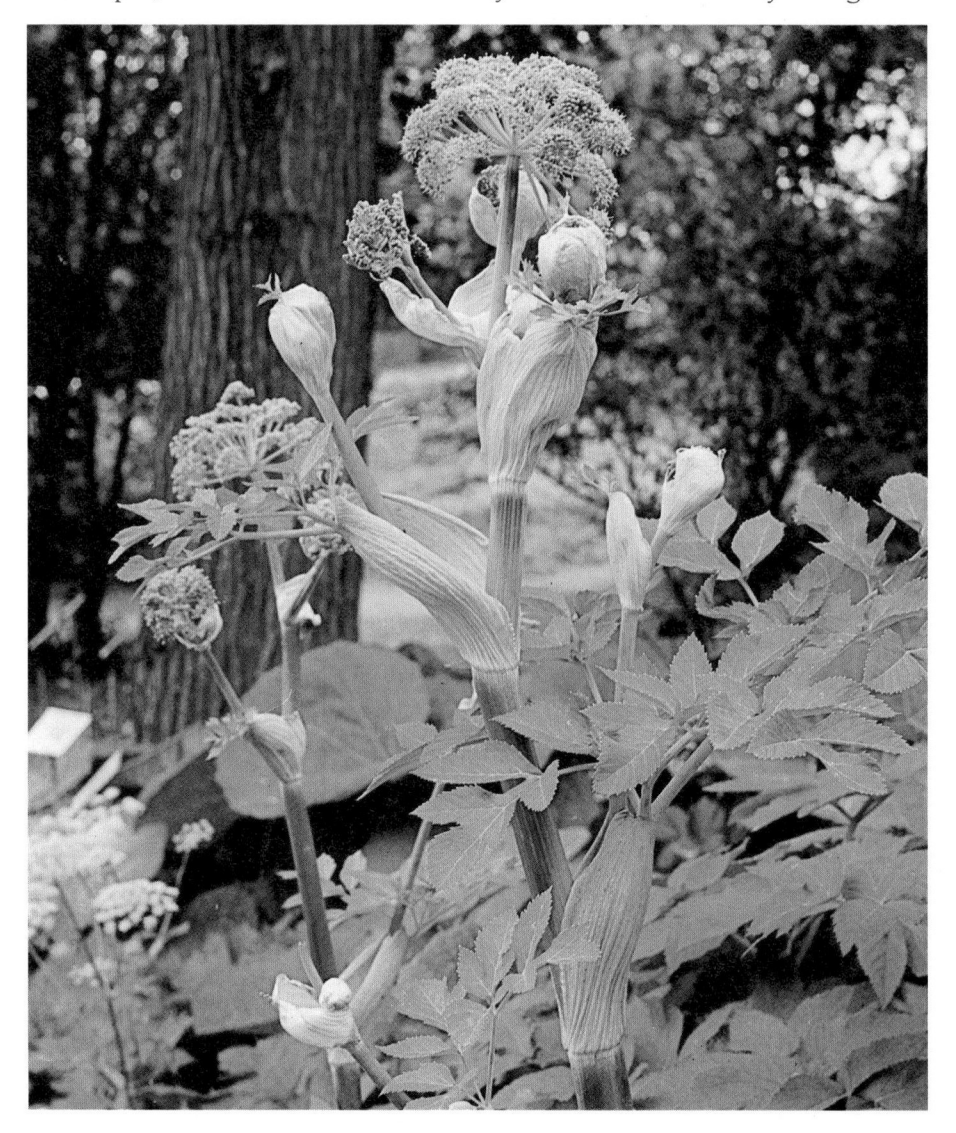

Angelica has always been highly valued for its health preserving properties. This tall, attractive plant can be used as the basis for a skin tonic, as a stimulating bath additive or as a breath freshener.

Angelica
(Angelica archangelica)

This plant is thought to have originated in Syria from where it spread to Europe. It has long enjoyed the place of honour at the forefront of all the known medicinal plants. The Vikings and Norsemen thought it to be of heavenly origin, and to this day the Dutch call it 'the plant of the Holy Ghost'. It arrived in Britain in the 16th century, and its name derives from the fact that Michael the Archangel appeared in a vision declaring that this herb could cure the plague. It was duly used to stave off the virulent plague of 1665. It was also believed to protect the wearer from witchcraft.

Description: A perennial which can grow to 1.8m (6ft) with a hollow fluted stem and large sheaths around the leaves. It has clusters of greenish white flowers and a pleasant aroma.

Collection: The roots should be dug up in autumn, the leaves picked in early summer.

Availability: Find it growing in meadows and along banks of streams. Packet seeds can be bought from garden centres, and the dried leaves and roots are sold at herbalists. Oil of Angelica can also be purchased, but it is very expensive.

Active constituents: Silica.

Cosmetic uses: As part of a stimulating bath mixture, and the root can be chewed to freshen the breath.

Balm
(Melissa officinalis)

The name comes from the Greek word *Melissa* for the honey bee, and it was thought that bees stayed in hives where balm grew nearby. Also known as Lemon balm because it exudes a lemon-like fragrance when pressed. The leaves were woven into garlands to wear at banquets when the air was oppressive, and women wore it in amulets of silk to promote love. It was also believed to renew youth, strengthen the brain and prevent baldness!

Description: A hardy perennial which grows up to 61cm (2ft) and has branching hairy stems with opposite leaves. White flowers grow in whorls on the leaf axils.

Collection: The leaves and aerial parts (all parts above ground) should be picked at the beginning of the flowering period.

Availability: This herb grows wild all over Europe, or can be grown from seeds.

Active constituents: Silica, tannins, organic acids.

Cosmetic uses: As a soothing bath additive.

Bay
(Laurus nobilis)

The ancient Romans had a great respect for bay. Its name comes from the verb *laudare* to praise, and generals crowned themselves with bay laurel when returning from victorious military campaigns. The Anglo-Saxon word for crown was *bay*. Roman Emperors wore bay during thunderstorms to ward off evil spirits. This plant has been cultivated in Britain since the 16th century, and has long been used to flavour food and for its antiseptic qualities.

Description: An evergreen shrub that can grow as high as 3.3m (10ft). It has shiny mid-green, aromatic leaves, and clusters of greenish-yellow flowers in spring.

Collection: The leaves can be picked at any time.

Availability: Frequently cultivated in parks and gardens. Small plants can be bought from nurseries. The dried leaves can be found at supermarkets, grocery stores and from most herbalists.

Active constituents: Volatile oil.

Cosmetic uses: As a soothing bath essence, an antiseptic and in perfumes.

Camomile, chamomile
(Anthemis nobilis)

There are several different species of camomile, all of which have similar properties. True camomile has been praised since ancient times for its healing qualities. The Egyptians dedicated it to the gods, and it has been a favourite with country folk for many centuries.

Description: A low-growing creeping plant with hairy, branching stems and feathery leaves. It has small yellow and white

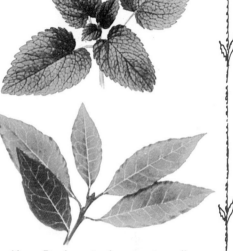

Above: Bay has a lovely aromatic smell when its leaves are rubbed between the fingers. It is used to make up different perfumes and is lovely when added to bath essence.

Top: Balm has a delightful lemony fragrance which is often used in perfumes. Added to the bath it makes a soothing and sweet smelling beauty aid.

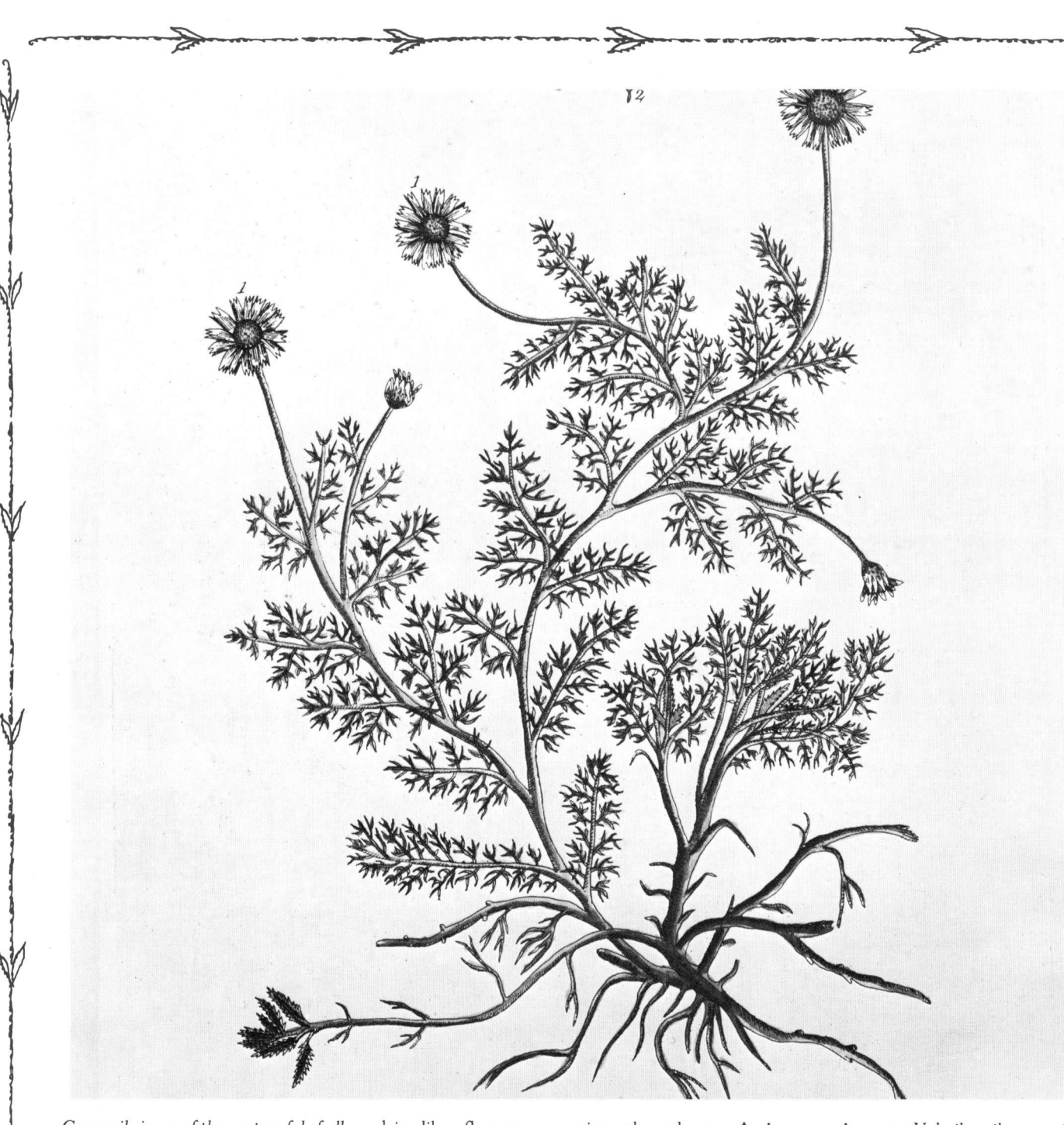

Camomile is one of the most useful of all herbs for cosmetic purposes. It is excellent for smoothing and lightening the skin in face creams and cleansers. It also has a very mild bleaching action on fair hair and adds a lovely shine.

daisy-like flowers appearing throughout summer.

Collection: The flowerheads should be picked at the start of the flowering season.

Availability: The plant grows wild on common land, or dried flowerheads can be bought from herbalists.

Active constituents: Volatile oil, organic acids.

Cosmetic uses: Camomile makes an excellent cleanser, especially for problem skins. It soothes inflammations and is a relaxing bath additive. Its most interesting cosmetic use is as a fair hair conditioner and lightener.

Clover
(Trifolium pratense)

Clover comes from the Latin *clava* meaning a club, and this is the symbol on playing cards. Red clover was used extensively by the Anglo-Saxons for its medicinal properties and to guard against witchcraft. The four-leaved foliage has always been considered a good luck charm. White clover (*Trifolium repens*) has similar properties.

Description: A perennial with stems up to 1.2m (4ft) high, it has red or white globe-like flowers.

Collection: Flowerheads at beginning of flowering season.

Availability: Clover grows wild in meadows and gardens, and is commonly found growing in lawns. Dried flowerheads can be bought from herbalists.

Active constituents: Silica and lime.

Cosmetic uses: A lightening hair rinse, a soothing cream and a mild bleach for freckles.

Comfrey
(Symphytum officinale)

This herb has been popular since the Middle Ages as a healing plant. Other names for it include Knitbone, Boneset and Knitback, as it was used to speed the mending of broken bones.

Description: A robust perennial with a branching stem and alternate hairy leaves, it can reach a height of 92cm (3ft). It has small, drooping bell-shaped creamy or purple flowers, which bloom throughout the summer months.

Collection: The root can be dug up in autumn, and the leaves and herbage at the start of the flowering season.

Availability: Comfrey grows wild in meadows, ditches and alongside streams. Small plants can be bought from nurseries, or the leaves and roots ready-dried from herbalists.

Active constituents: A substantial amount of allantoin, silica, tannins.

Cosmetic uses: Its emollient action makes it a perfect addition to body lotions and soaps, hand creams and hair conditioners.

Cornflower
(Centaurea cyanus)

This was the favourite flower of the Roman goddess Flora, and the name Centaurea is derived from the Centaur Chiron who taught man the healing virtues of herbs. This was a favourite garden flower in Tudor times, and the blue dye from the flowers was used to colour linen, and as a pigment for watercolours. The flower was also considered a lucky charm.

Description: A hardy annual and upright plant which can grow up to 92cm (3ft). It has long narrow leaves and brilliant blue flowers.

Collection: The flowers should be picked at the start of the flowering season.

Availability: Cornflowers used to grow profusely in meadows and on waste ground but have been greatly reduced by the use of modern fertilizers. Seeds and young plants are sold at gardening centres. The dried flowerheads can be bought from larger herbalists.

Active constituents: Silica.

Cosmetic uses: Cornflowers make a soothing bath for tired, swollen eyes, and are a useful addition to eye make-up remover and eye creams. They are also good to add to facial steaming mixtures.

Cowslip
(Primula veris)

The Anglo Saxons called this plant *cuslippe* which means cow's breath – a reference to the flower's distinctive smell. In old herbals it is often referred to as Herb Peter and Key Flower, as the flowers were thought to resemble the Keys of Heaven which St. Peter holds. Cowslip has been used since earliest times to treat skin problems and nervous complaints, and to take away spots, wrinkles and freckles. It was also thought to strengthen the brain.

Description: The leaves lie close to the ground in a rosette from which the stalk rises, topped by creamy-yellow flowers.

Collection: The flowers should be gathered at the beginning of the flowering period.

Availability: The cowslip has become in-

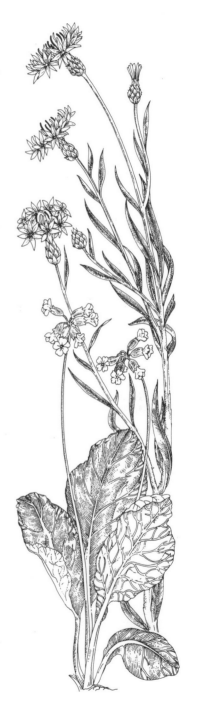

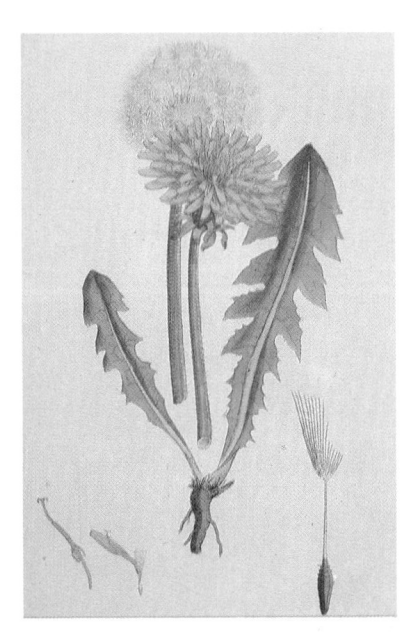

Dandelions are one of the most readily available herbs as they are abundant in the wild. They exude a richly emollient latex juice which is very soothing to dry skin in cleansing milks and also in moisturizing lotions.

creasingly rare as a wild plant, but is still quite widespread in Ireland. The dried flowerheads can be bought from herbalists.
Active constituents: Saponins, silica, tannins.
Cosmetic uses: Beneficial in all face creams and sunburn lotions.

Dandelion
(Taraxacum officinale)

The name derives from the Greek *taraxos* – a disorder, and *akos*, remedy. Legend has it that the dandelion was born of the dust raised by the chariot of the sun. Magicians thought highly of its magic properties – rubbing yourself all over with it would make you welcome everywhere, and able to obtain whatever you wished. It became known as *Dent de Lion* (Lion's Tooth) because of its serrated leaves. Young women used to blow away the seed heads to see how many years they would have to wait for a husband, and blowing a dandelion 'clock' is a traditional game to tell the time.
Description: The plant has serrated green leaves and a tapering root (no stem) which exudes a milky latex juice when cut. Throughout the summer the plant bears bright yellow, flat-topped flowers with numerous tiny petals.
Collection: The root should be dug up in autumn or early spring and, the herbage picked in spring.
Availability: Dandelions grow wild everywhere throughout Europe, particularly on wasteland and grass verges. The roots and herbage can be bought from herbalists.
Active constituents: Resin, gluten, potassium.
Cosmetic uses: Cleansing milks and moisturizers.

Elder
(Sambucus nigra)

A wealth of superstition surrounds this tree, often thought of as a symbol of grief. It was believed that Judas was hanged on an elder tree, and even that the Cross of Calvary was made of it. As a result, elder became the emblem of sorrow and death, and gypsies

will not use it as firewood. It was also considered unwise to make furniture from it. The flowers, however, have long been used as an aid to beauty.
Description: The tree can grow up to 10m (32ft). It has dark green leaves, a greyish-green bark and small creamy-white flowers which grow to form a wide plate. They have a strong, sickly perfume. These flowers are followed by clusters of black berries in autumn.
Collection: The flowers should be cut off with short stalks at the beginning of the flowering period.
Availability: The elder grows on open land and in gardens throughout Europe. The dried flowers are available from herbalists.
Active constituents: Organic acids, silica, tannins, mineral salts, amines.
Cosmetic uses: Elderflower water appeared on every lady's dressing table for hundreds of years, as it has great powers to whiten and soften the skin. It can be used in moisturizers and cleansing milks, hand and body lotions, and to bleach freckles, particularly in the summer months.

Eucalyptus
(Eucalyptus globulus)

A native of Australia and Tasmania, this tree was widely known as the Fever Tree as it was cultivated in swampy areas for its antiseptic qualities which helped to fight against malaria and typhoid. The oil from its leaves has long been used in medicine.
Description: A tree with leathery, blue-green leaves which are studded with glands containing the fragrant volatile oil. The flowers are covered by a cup-like membrane which is thrown off as the flower begins to expands.
Collection: The leaves are picked at beginning of the flowering season.
Availability: Young shrubs can be bought from gardening centres, the dried leaves can be found at herbalists.
Active constituents: The essential oil of Eucalyptus.
Cosmetic uses: It is a refreshing bath additive, a mouthwash and an effective remedy for sunburn.

Fennel
(Foeniculum vulgare)

The ancient Greeks and Romans were great believers in the powers of fennel, believing it strengthened the body and the eyesight, and helped with slimming. In mediaeval times it was hung over doors to warn off evil spirits, especially on Midsummer's Eve. People put it in their keyholes to ensure their sleep was undisturbed by ghosts and gremlins.

Description: Fennel is a perennial with an erect branching stem and blue-green, feathery foliage. In summer it produces clusters of brilliant yellow flowers. It can reach 1.5m (5ft).

Collection: The leaves at the start of the flowering period, the seeds when the fruits are ripe.

Availability: Growing plants are often found near the sea, and small plants can be bought from garden centres. Dried leaves and seeds can be bought from herbalists and health food shops.

Active constituents: Silica, oil, organic acids and proteins.

Cosmetic uses: The leaves can be used in facial cleansers and steam treatments, they also make a good hair conditioner. Fennel seeds sweeten the breath when they are chewed.

Houseleek
(Sempervivum tectorum)

The ancient Greeks and Romans dedicated this plant to Zeus (Jupiter) as it was thought to resemble his beard. They believed the plant could guard a house against thunder and lightning. Later in the 9th century AD King Charlemagne ordered that it should be planted on the rooftops.

Description: A hardy evergreen with a rosette of fleshy green leaves, the purple edges fringed with hairs. In summer, small pink daisy-like flowers appear on tall stems.

Collection: The leaves before flowering period.

Availability: This is a common garden plant, often growing in walls and on roofs. Small plants and seeds are available from nurseries. The dried leaves can be bought from herbalists.

Active constituents: Malic acid and also some lime.

Cosmetic uses: Very beneficial to the skin in creams, lotions and cleansing steam treatments.

Hyssop
(Hyssopus officinalis)

This Greek name derives from azob (a holy herb) as it was used for cleaning sacred places.

Description: An evergreen bushy herb which can grow to 61cm (2ft) with square stems and flowers in whorls, coloured blue, red or white.

Collection: The flowerheads and also the leaves at the beginning of the flowering season.

Availability: Can be grown from small plants or seeds. It is also commonly found growing wild all over Europe. Dried flowers and leaves can also be bought from herbalist shops.

Active constituents: Volatile oil.

Cosmetic uses: A good cleanser for acne, and as a bath additive to relieve aches and pains.

Ivy, common
(Hedera helix)

Ivy was held in high esteem by the ancient Romans, and was regarded as an antidote to drunkenness, which is why Bacchus is always shown with a wreath of ivy. Poets wore crowns of the plant, and Greek priests gave a wreath of ivy to all couples on their wedding day as it was regarded as the emblem of fidelity.

Description: An evergreen climber with glossy dark-green leaves.

Collection: The leaves in spring.

Availability: Ivy grows profusely on hedges, banks and ditches and it often appears all over buildings.

Active constituents: Astringents.

Cosmetic uses: As a stimulating bath additive, a foot bath, an anti-cellulite cream, and to relieve sunburn.

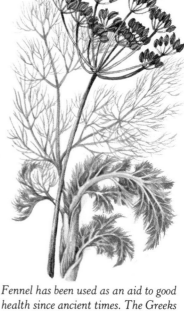

Fennel has been used as an aid to good health since ancient times. The Greeks chewed the seeds to sweeten the breath and to help stave off the appetite when they were trying to slim. The leaves are very stimulating in facial steaming treatments, and they make a good hair conditioner.

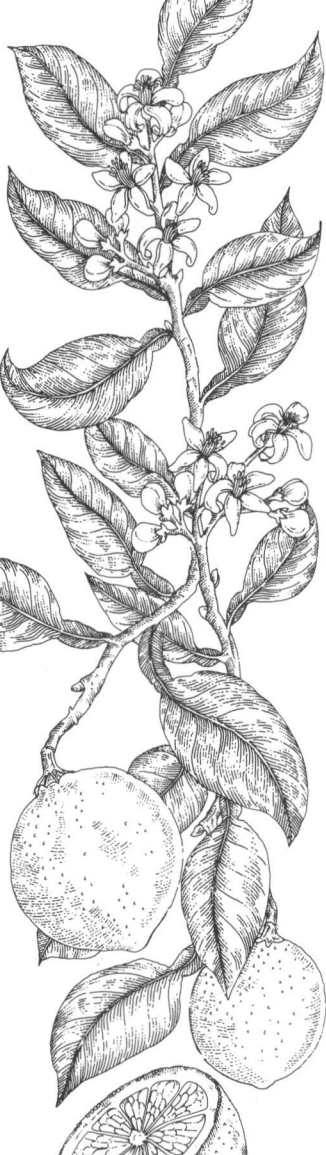

Lavender
(Lavendula spica)

The name originates from the Latin *lavare* meaning to wash. Lavender has been used since ancient times as a fragrant cleanser. Because of its antiseptic qualities it was also used to spray beds to get rid of bedbugs, and to keep the hair free of lice. In Elizabethan times a laundress was known as a *lavendre* because it was usual to wash clothes in lavender water.

Description: A silver-leaved woody shrub with spiky mauve flowers and a highly distinctive fragrance.

Collection: The flower stalks and flowers in mid-summer when flowers are full.

Availability: A common garden shrub, it can be grown from seed or small plants. Dried flowers are available from herbalists.

Active constituents: A volatile oil containing linalool and linalyl acetate.

Cosmetic uses: As a fragrant oil or toilet water it can also be added to creams, skin tonics and cleansers, bath soaks and soaps.

Lime, Linden
(Tilia europaea)

Dedicated to Venus, the lime has always been valuable both in medicine and beauty preparations. Saint Hildegard warded off the plague in the Middle Ages with lime blossom worn in a ring.

Description: A smooth straight tree, growing to 9m (30ft). It has mid-green heart-shaped leaves, and yellowish-white flowers, hanging in clusters. The blooms have a sweet fragrance, and bees produce a fine honey from them.

Collection: The flowers before they reach full bloom.

Availability: Lime grows in many parks and gardens, and wild throughout Europe. The dried flowers can be bought from herbalists.

Active constituents: Volatile oil, organic acids, silica, vitamins.

Cosmetic uses: As a skin lotion for refining the skin, as a moisturizer and to bleach freckles. Also a hair conditioning rinse, and a soothing bath additive.

Marigold
(Calendula officinalis)

This flower received its botanical name because it flowers on the first day (the calends) of most months of the year. A native of southern Europe, it has been in use for hundreds of years as a healing plant. In the American Civil War it was widely used as an antiseptic to clean wounds. The leaves helped to reduce fevers.

Collection: The flowers before they reach full bloom.

Description: A hardy annual which has orange flowers and pale green leaves.

Availability: Marigolds grow wild and in gardens, and can be grown from seeds or young plants from garden centres. The dried flowers can be bought from herbalists.

Active constituents: Antiseptics.

Cosmetic uses: As moisturizers, cleansers and skin tonics for problem skin. Also as a lightening rinse for light brown hair.

Marshmallow
(Althea officinalis)

The name derives from the Greek *athos* – a cure. They regarded it as a general cure-all, while the Romans enjoyed it as a vegetable.

Description: The marshmallow has grey-green serrated, alternate leaves, and large, cup-shaped, light-pink flowers. The erect stems may grow as high as 1.2m (4ft) and the whole plant is covered with a velvety down.

Collection: The leaves should be picked in mid-summer, when the flowers are just coming into bloom and the roots gathered in spring or autumn.

Availability: This plant grows by ponds and streams, and on salt marshes. It can be found throughout Britain and Europe. Both the dried root and leaves can be bought from herbalists.

Active constituents: Starch, mucilage, pectin, oil.

Cosmetic uses: Marshmallow has fine emollient and skin softening properties, so it is used in many skin lotions and creams for dry skins. The leaves can also be used as an eye wash.

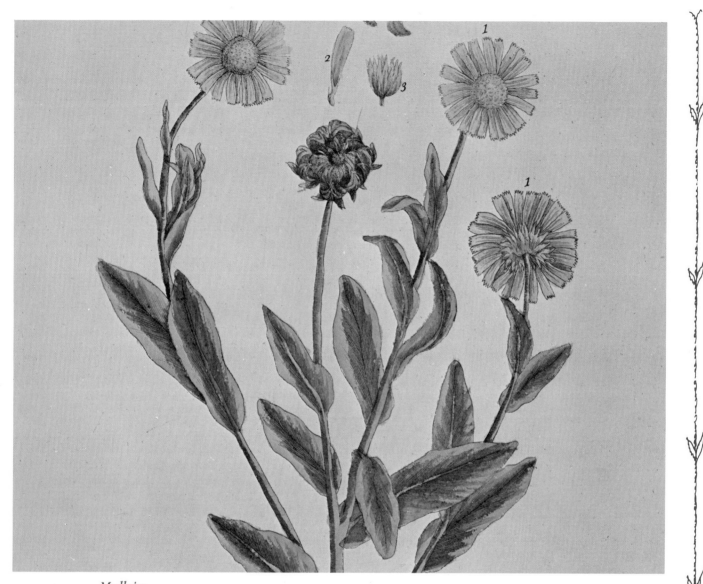

Mullein
(Verbascum thapsus)

Another name for this plant is Torches, as the leaves and stems make excellent tinder when very dry. An old superstition says that witches used lamps made of these wicks in their spells. In both Europe and Asia it was believed to be capable of driving out evil spirits. Poor people used to fill their stockings with the leaves to keep their feet warm.

Description: A biennial, with a basal rosette of leaves forming during the first year from which the flower stalk grows in the second, growing as high as 92cm (3ft). The yellow flowers form in clusters throughout the summer.

Collection: The flowers are collected as they open.

Availability: Mullein grows wild on waste ground throughout Europe. It can be bought dried from herb shops.

Active constituents: Mucilage, starch, sugars, pectins, mineral salts.

Cosmetic uses: The yellow flowers provide a golden lightener for the hair.

Marigold is renowned for its antiseptic and healing properties, so it is invaluable in tonics, cleansers and moisturizers for problem skins. It can also be used to impart a golden shine to blonde or light-brown hair.

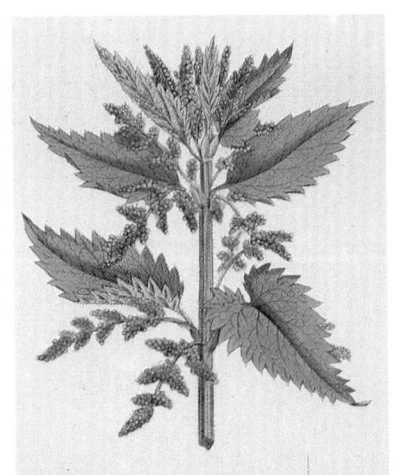

Above: Nettle may be a plant children learn to avoid because of its painful stinging action, but it is highly beneficial in hair products for problems such as greasy hair and dandruff. It also makes a very good skin tonic.

Below: Parsley is a very common culinary herb which also makes an ideal breath freshener when chewed after eating foods containing garlic. It is often added to skin and hair tonics, and an infusion of parsley can help to fade noticeable freckles.

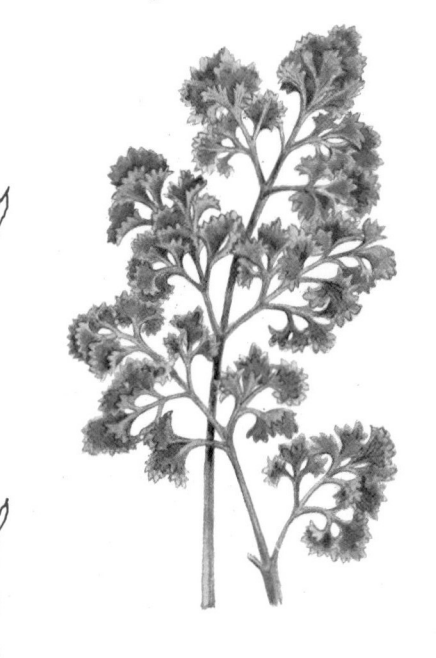

Nettle
(Urtica diocia)

The name nettle comes from the Anglo-Saxon *naoedl* meaning needle – alluding to the painful stinging action of the plant. Also from *net* meaning an item that has been spun. The thread made from the hairs of the plant was used extensively in Scandinavia and Scotland. It was also believed to have magic properties – it was thought to quell fear if held in the hand with sprigs of yarrow. It has long been used in medicines for its high vitamin C content.

Description: A perennial with erect stems growing to 1.5m (5ft). The stem has pairs of dark green leaves, and the whole plant is covered with stinging hairs. It produces thin catkins of tiny green flowers from June to September.

Collection: The aerial parts before flowering, but only the leafy young tops of the plant.

Availability: Nettles grow abundantly on waste ground throughout Europe. The dried leaves can be bought from herbalists.

Active constituents: Mineral salts, vitamins.

Cosmetic uses: A skin tonic and bath soak, also a hair rinse for greasy hair and an anti-dandruff treatment.

Parsley
(Petroselinum crispum)

There are many strange superstitions attached to parsley. It is said to be very bad luck to try and transplant it, and it is thought to have to go seven times to the devil and return to its place before it can grow. It was used in funeral rites by the Greeks, and they believed it sprang from the spilled blood of Archemorous, the great hero. The champions of the Isthmian games were crowned with garlands of parsley.

Description: A hardy biennial, it has bright green curled foliage and greenish-yellow flowers in summer.

Collection: The aerial parts.

Availability: Seeds and young plants can be bought from nurseries, the fresh cut herb from greengrocers. The dried leaves can be bought from supermarkets, delicatessens and health food shops.

Active constituents: Iron, calcium, vitamins.

Cosmetic uses: As a lotion for troubled skins, an anti-freckle treatment, as a hair rinse and to alleviate dandruff. It is also a well-known breath freshener, especially if chewed after eating garlic.

Peppermint
(Mentha piperita)

The Greeks used peppermint in perfume, the Romans enjoyed it in their wine, while the women chewed it to sweeten the breath. Students wore garlands of peppermint as it was thought to be good for the mind, and it was frequently strewn on floors for the aromatic smell and placed in beds to keep linen smelling fresh.

Description: The stems grow up to 1.2m (4ft) high, with leaves that are finely serrated and slightly hairy underneath. The flowers grow in whorls of violet-coloured blooms in the axils of the upper leaves.

Collection: The leaves and stems, before the flowering period.

Availability: Grows profusely in gardens and in the wild. Nurseries have young plants, the dried leaves can be bought at grocery shops and from herbalists.

Active constituents: Volatile oil, menthol.

Cosmetic uses: A complexion milk for problem skin, a refreshing skin tonic, cologne, a stimulating bath additive, a gargle and mouthwash.

Pine
(Pinus)

There are many different species, with similar properties. The ancient Egyptians used the turpentine from the resin for many ailments, and it has been employed in making varnishes. Pine resins have been used to make paints and soaps.

Description: Pines usually have straight unbranching trunks, with needle-like leaves. They are evergreens and highly aromatic.

Collection: The pine needles at any time, and the green cones.

Availability: Pines grow in woodland and forests throughout Europe. Available dried from herbalists.
Active constituents: Resins, organic acids, turpentine.
Cosmetic uses: Bath soaks, hair rinse.

Rose
(Rosa)

The most prized and precious of all flowers, it is valued as much for its uses as its beauty. The rose used to adorn the shields of Persian warriors, and the first cultivated roses probably originated in Persia. They were pure red and strongly perfumed. The Romans were very attached to roses – they were suspended above the table at political meetings to ensure confidentiality. The modern ceiling rose is a legacy. It is thought that the rose was introduced into England by the Romans, where it carried on its reputation for inspiring love and purity.
Description: A shrubby perennial with small dark green leaves and brilliantly coloured and perfumed petals. The perfection of the flower makes it the most famous flower in the world.
Collection: The petals, before the flower reaches full bloom.
Availability: Roses grow prolifically throughout British gardens, and small shrubs can be bought from garden centres. The dried petals can be bought from herbalists, but it is most commonly bought as an oil or water.
Active constituents: Volatile oil, tannic acid and resin.
Cosmetic uses: Perfumes, colognes, skin cleansers, moisturizers and toners, hand and body lotions, mouthwashes.

Rosemary
(Rosmarinus officinalis)

This herb takes its name from *rosmarinus* – rose of the sea, because it was often found near sea shores. In Ancient Greece it was thought to refresh the mind and gladden the spirits, and students wore it in their hair to improve their learning abilities. Rosemary bushes were planted on either side of doorways to perfume the clothes of those who brushed past. It was also used at funerals to keep the memory of the departed 'green', and Napoleon used large quantities of Rosemary eau-de-cologne when he was weary after battle. The herb is thought to have arrived in Britain in the 14th century, when it was used as incense.
Description: An evergreen shrub with mid-green leathery leaves that turn under at the edges, the undersides are covered with fine white hairs. The plant can grow to 2m (6½ft) and the lilac-coloured flowers appear in whorls in small clusters in the axils of the leaves, blooming from spring until autumn.
Collection: The leaves and aerial parts in the flowering season.
Availability: Rosemary grows profusely in Mediterranean countries. It can be cultivated from small plants sold at nurseries. The dried herb is frequently used in cooking, so is easily obtained from supermarkets, grocery shops and herbalists.
Active constituents: Silica, tannins, saponins, organic acids.
Cosmetic uses: A facial steam treatment, a foot and bath soak, as an anti-dandruff preparation and a hair rinse.

Sage
(Salvia officinalis)

The ancient Romans called sage, *salvia*, meaning health and salvation, as it was believed to give long life to all who used it. It was thought to be good for the brain, senses and memory. In Europe, it has long been used to whiten the teeth.
Description: A hardy perennial, evergreen shrub with a woody stem and oval, grey-green wrinkled leaves. Violet flowers in clusters appear from early to mid-summer.
Collection: The leaves and aerial parts before flowering.
Availability: Sage is cultivated throughout Europe and North America. Small plants and seeds can be bought from garden centres, the dried herb at most supermarkets, grocers and herbalists.
Active constituents: Silica, tannins, vitamins, resins.
Cosmetic uses: In soaps and perfumes, bath

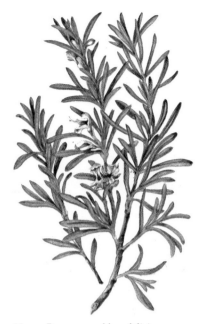

Above: Rosemary adds a delicious fragrance to bath soaks and makes an aromatic cologne. It also helps combat dandruff in hair rinses.

Below: Sage has numerous beneficial qualities. The leaves can be chewed on their own to remove teeth stains and infusions of the herb make ideal skin tonics and hair rinses.

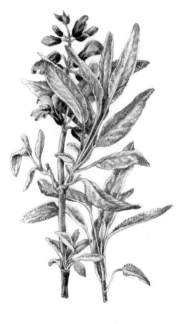

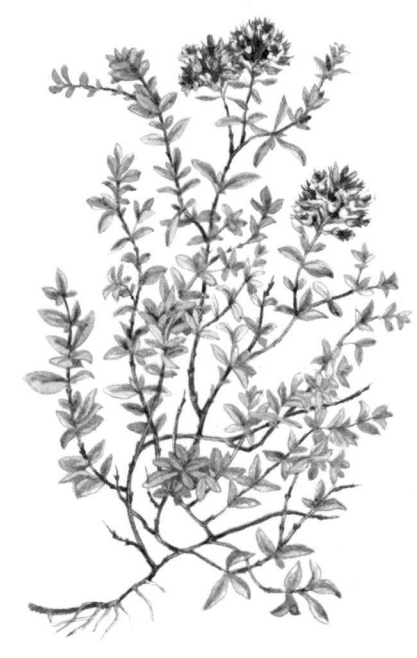

Thyme has long been used in times of war to help disinfect wounds, and its highly aromatic properties make it a delightful addition to baths and foot soaks. Its antiseptic qualities make it a useful base for facial astringents, and an infusion of thyme works well to soothe an itchy scalp.

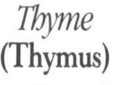

soaks and mouth washes, toothpastes and lip salves. Also in shampoos.

Soapwort
(Saponaria officinalis)

The generic name, *saponaria,* comes from the Latin *sapo* meaning soap, because the leaves and stems placed in water make a creamy cleansing lather. People first washed their bodies and their clothes by crushing and making an infusion of the leaves. The juice was also believed to speed healing.

Description: A hardy annual with erect stems which branch at the top, it can reach 1.2m (4ft). It has large, elongated leaves and clusters of pink or white flowers.

Collection: The roots should be dug up in early spring or autumn, the aerial parts collected at the beginning of the flowering period.

Availability: Grows widely in damp places such as the banks of rivers and damp meadows. The dried herb can be bought from herbalists.

Active constituents: Saponins, flavones.

Cosmetic uses: In body and hair shampoos.

Tansy
(Tanacetum vulgare)

The name derives from the Greek word for immortality. This is thought to be because it had excellent preserving qualities when used on corpses. It was often used as a strewing herb indoors because it kept flies away. Tansy cakes were eaten after Lent, and these cakes, known as Tansies, came to be eaten on Easter Day in remembrance of the bitter herbs eaten by the Jews at Passover.

Description: A perennial growing to 92cm (3ft) it has aromatic dark green, ferny leaves and clusters of small yellow flowers.

Collection: The leaves picked before the flowering period.

Availability: Tansy grows wild and in gardens, and can be grown from seeds. The dried leaves can be bought from herbalists.

Active constituents: Tanacetin, tannic acid, volatile oil.

Cosmetic uses: As an additive to facial steaming mixtures, as a bath soak.

Thyme
(Thymus)

The name derives from the Greek *thumos* meaning sacrifical smoke, as this herb was often burnt during ancient sacrifices and in places of worship. The Romans used it in their baths and brought it to Britain where it has been cultivated since the 15th century. In war time it has been widely used to disinfect and clean wounds, and with sage and rosemary has more uses than any of the other herbs.

Description: An evergreen shrub with a creeping woody stem and deep green, aromatic leaves, bearing small clusters of small mauve flowers.

Collection: Flowers and aerial parts at the beginning of the flowering period.

Availability: It can be found growing abundantly in fields, or purchased as young plants from nurseries. Larger greengrocers keep fresh sprigs, and it can be bought dried from supermarkets and grocers.

Active constituents: Silica, thymol, tannins, organic acids.

Cosmetic uses: Astringent face tonics, a bath additive, a foot balm, shampoo and anti-dandruff lotion.

Valerian
(Valeriana officinalis)

This herb takes its name from the Latin *valere,* meaning to be well. In medieval times it was regarded as a cure-all, and was used in many medicines and perfumes. It was also used as a cure for epilepsy.

Description: A robust herb with bright green, feathery leaves on stems that can reach up to 92cm (3ft). It has clusters of tiny pink flowers in early summer.

Collection: The root is dug up in autumn and dried.

Availability: Valerian is found growing wild in ditches, by river banks and near seas and marshland. The root is the only part used, and is sold by herbalists.

Active constituents: Silica, esters, organic acids, alkaloids.

Cosmetic uses: A soothing bath soak, and as a lotion for acned skins.

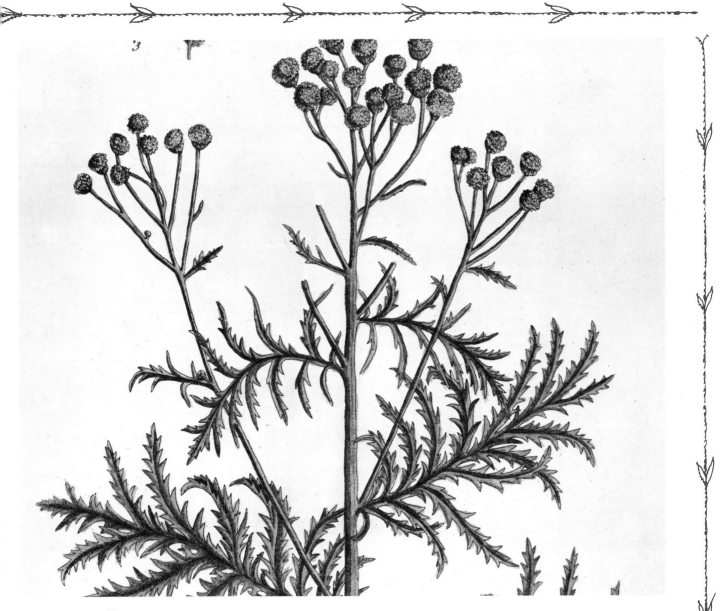

Yarrow
(Achillea millefolium)

The Greek generic name derives from its connection with Achilles who is said to have used yarrow to tend his soldiers' wounds. It was called the Military Herb by the ancients. It was also dedicated to the Devil by witches, and used in their spells. Some yarrow sewn up in flannel and placed under the pillow was supposed to bring a vision of the sleeper's future spouse. It was even thought to allay baldness when rubbed on the scalp.

Description: A perennial with erect stalk, branching at the top, that can reach 61cm (2ft). It has feathery foliage and clusters of white or pink daisy-like flowers.

Collection: The aerial parts of the plant at the beginning of the flowering season.

Availability: Yarrow can be found growing wild by roadsides and in barren, sandy places. The dried herb is available from herbalists.

Active constituents: Silica, tannins, mineral salts.

Cosmetic uses: Cleansers, hair rinses.

Tansy was used by the ancients for preserving corpses, and was often strewn indoors to keep the air fresh. It has a stimulating and astringent action on the skin when used in facial steaming treatments and bath soaks.

Growing Guide for Herbs and Flowers	Popular name	Latin name	Description
	Angelica	*Angelica archangelica*	Hardy biennial or short-lived perennial. Maximum growth 1.8m (6ft)
	Balm	*Melissa officinalis*	Perennial. Maximum growth 61cm (2ft)
	Bay	*Laurus nobilis*	Evergreen. Maximum growth 3m (10ft)
	Camomile	*Anthemis nobilis*	Hardy annual. Maximum growth 30cm (12in)
	Clover	*Trifolium pratense*	Perennial. Maximum growth 1.2m (4ft)
	Comfrey	*Symphytum officinale*	Perennial. Maximum growth 92cm (3ft)
	Cornflower	*Centaurea cyanus*	Annual. Maximum growth 92cm (3ft)
	Eucalyptus	*Eucaluptus globulus*	Evergreen. Maximum growth 3m (10ft)
	Fennel	*Foeniculum vulgare*	Perennial. Maximum growth 1.5m (5ft)
	Houseleek.	*Sempervivum tectorum*	Evergreen succulent. Maximum growth 15cm (6in)
	Hyssop	*Hyssopus officinalis*	Evergreen. Maximum growth 61cm (2ft)
	Lavender	*Lavendula spica*	Perennial. Maximum growth 1.2m (4ft)
	Marigold	*Calendula officinalis*	Annual. Maximum growth 50cm (20in)
	Marshmallow	*Althaea officinalis*	Perennial. Maximum growth 1.2m (4ft)
	Mullein	*Verbascum thapsus*	Biennial. Maximum growth 92cm (3ft)
	Parsley	*Petroselinum crispum*	Biennial. Maximum growth 30cm (12in)
	Peppermint	*Mentha piperita*	Perennial. Maximum growth 1.2m (4ft)
	Rose	*Rosa*	Perennial
	Rosemary	*Rosmarinus officinalis*	Evergreen. Maximum growth 2m (6½ft)
	Sage	*Salvia officinalis*	Evergreen. Maximum growth 61cm (2ft)
	Tansy	*Tanacetum vulgare*	Perennial. Maximum growth 92cm (3ft)
	Thyme	*Thymus*	Evergreen. Maximum growth 30cm (12in)
	Valerian	*Valeriana officinalis*	Perennial. Maximum growth 92cm (3ft)
	Yarrow	*Achillea millefolium*	Perennial. Maximum growth 6cm (2ft)

Planting and cultivation	Container growing
Sow seeds in March/April in shady position and moist rich soil. Replant seedlings 25cm (10in) apart. The mature plant will seed itself, leaving you to replant seedlings.	Not suitable.
Sow seeds in spring in ordinary well-drained garden soil, ideally in a sunny position. Thin seedlings out to 30cm (12in) apart. In October cut growth back to just above ground level.	Can be grown in large pots using John Innes No 2 or 3.
Plant small plants in March/April in a sunny, sheltered position and ordinary garden soil. Pinch out new shoots to shape growing bush.	Can be grown in tubs, using John Innes No 3 potting compost.
Sow seeds in rows at 23cm (9in) intervals, or plant rooted cuttings or seedlings 15cm (6in) apart in March/April in a well-drained soil and sunny position. Tall plants may need supporting with twigs.	Can be grown in window boxes or tubs using John Innes potting compost Nos 2 or 3.
Plant in spring in a well-drained soil in a sunny position. (Shaded sites produce paler leaves).	Not suitable
Sow seeds in spring, plant small plants in autumn or spring, in ordinary damp garden soil, in sunny or shaded position. Cut back to basal growth after flowering.	Not suitable
Sow seeds in September or March. Thin out seedlings in a fertile well-drained soil, sunny position. Support taller stems with sticks.	Grows well in large pots, use John Innes No 2 or 3.
Plant young shrubs in early summer in a well-drained fertile soil, in a sunny position.	Grows well in large tubs – use John Innes No 1.
Sow seeds in shallow drills 5cm (2in) deep in spring in well-drained soil, sunny position. Thin seedlings to 40cm (16in) apart. Cut down in autumn to 10cm (4in).	Grows well in large tubs or window boxes, use John Innes No 2.
Plant small plants or seeds in spring or autumn in a well-drained ordinary soil, and in a sunny position.	Plant in medium pots with equal parts, John Innes potting compost No 2 and coarse sand.
Sow seeds in spring, small plants in spring or autumn. Likes a well-drained ordinary garden soil, sunny position. Transplant seedlings to 30cm (12in).	Grows well in large pots, use John Innes No 1.
Seeds take a long time to grow, so start with young plants in a well-drained limy soil and an open sunny position. Set plants 30cm (12in) apart, plant in spring or autumn.	Grows well in large tubs and window boxes in a sandy soil mix.
Sow seeds in spring then thin seedlings to 45cm (18in) or put in young plants in ordinary garden soil, sunny position. Plant will then re-seed itself.	Both seeds and plants grow well in pots and baskets using John Innes No 2 or 3.
Sow seeds in spring, re-plant seedlings 5cm (2in) apart in moist soil.	Not suitable
Sow seeds in spring, re-plant seedlings 30cm (12in) apart. Likes an ordinary well-drained garden soil, sunny position. Tall plants will need supporting. Cut down in November.	Not suitable
Sow seeds in spring and water well. Thin seedlings to 8cm (3in) and then to 20cm (8in) so they do not touch. Or put in young plants in spring. Likes a moist but well-drained soil, and semi-shade. Water and weed regularly, protect from frost.	Grows well in deep pots as it has long roots. Use John Innes No 2 or 3.
Plant young plants in spring or autumn – control spreading by restricting roots in a clay pot or bucket sunk in the earth. Likes moist soil, sun or partial shade. Pinch out flower buds to maintain maximum leaf growth.	Grows well in large pots or window boxes in moist soil. Use John Innes No 2 or 3.
Plant small shrubs according to the strain – basic provisions are good drainage, an open sunny position and plenty of water. Any soil except chalk. Plant in October to April, at least 61cm (2ft) apart.	Not suitable
Growing from seed is very slow so use small plants. Plant them in spring 45cm (18in) apart, in well-drained soil, sunny, sheltered position. Prune new shoots after flowering, protect from frost.	A good pot plant. Keep indoors in winter and clip into shape.
Sow seeds in spring, or small plants placed 40cm (16in) apart in well-hoed soil with good drainage. Sunny position. Prune regularly.	Grows well in large pots and window boxes. Use John Innes potting compost No 2 or 3.
Sow seeds in spring in ordinary garden soil, sunny position.	Not suitable
Sow seeds or young plants in spring in light, well-drained soil, sunny position. Trim tops after flowering to keep plants bushy. Re-plant every 3 years, protect from frost.	Grows well indoors in pots or in window boxes. Use John Innes No 2 or 3.
Sow seeds in spring, ordinary soil will do but prefers rich heavy loam. Likes a sunny position.	Not suitable
Plant between October and March in a well-drained garden soil, in a sunny position. Cut back to the ground in November.	Not suitable

An A to Z of organic ingredients

All the following fruits, nuts, vegetables and other natural ingredients have a long history as beauty aids and they are all included in the detailed recipe sections. They are all comparatively cheap to buy and easy to find, and making your own cosmetic preparations is an ideal way to use up any old fruits that are well past their best.

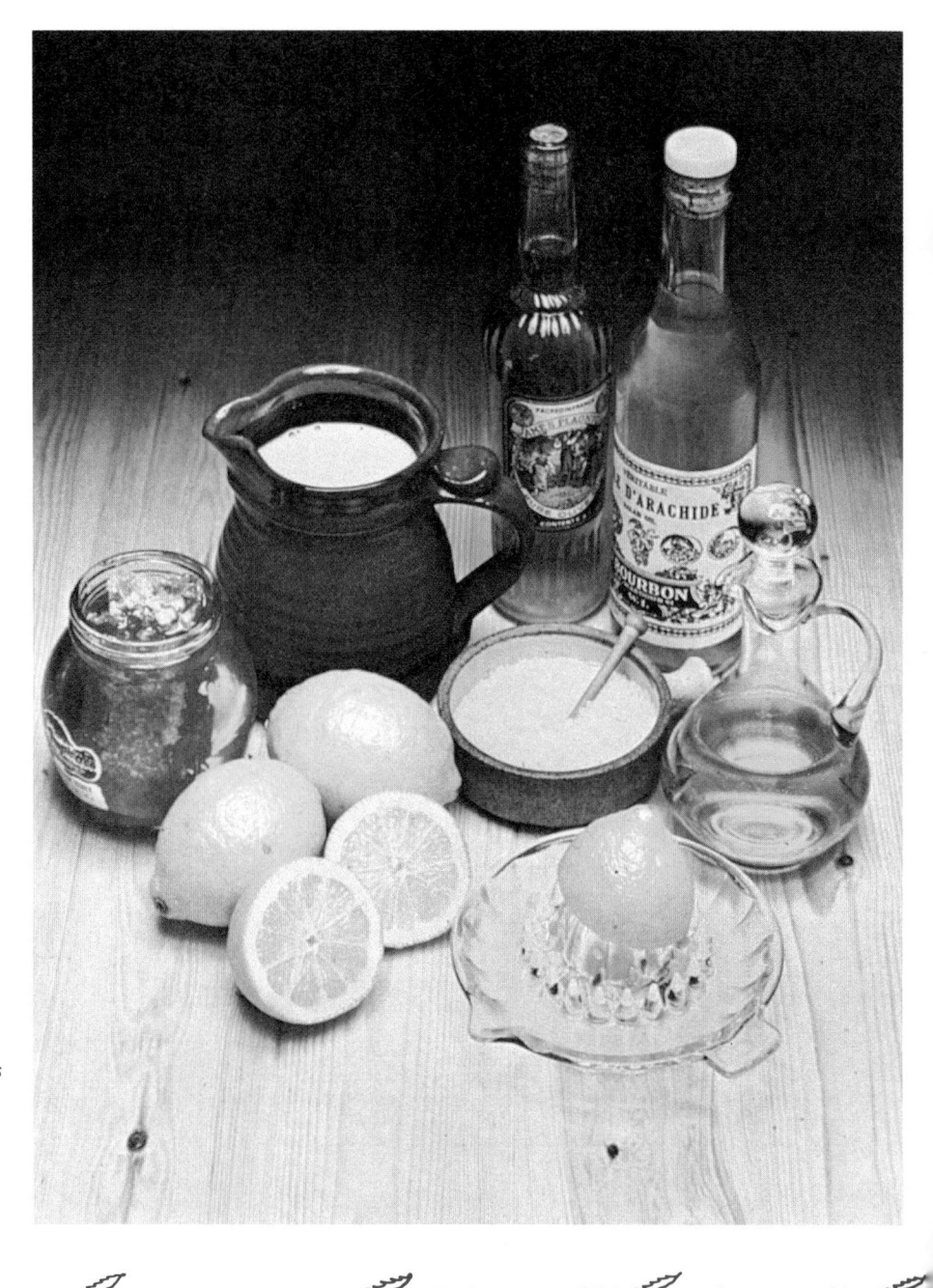

Many items that are perfect beauty aids can be found inside the kitchen cupboard. Do not discard the peels of vegetables and rinds of fruits when cooking, but keep them to use in your cosmetics.

Almond

Almond trees have always been loved for their beautiful blossoms, and the oil from the nuts is one of the most valuable cosmetics. The nuts can be pounded in water to extract a milky juice that makes an excellent cleansing milk, and the extracted oil is a rich and soothing addition to moisturizers. Almond oil makes a perfect base for many preparations.

Apple

According to legend this is the first fruit of the world and a great health provider. There are countless different varieties available today, from the rosy Cox's Orange Pippin to the yellow Golden Delicious. Apples are high in mineral salts and have more phosphates than any other fruit. They have been used as an aid to beauty since ancient times, and are ideal for fragrant skin tonics, masks and hair rinses.

Apricot

Apricots originated in China and Armenia, where reports were made of people living to over 150 years of age on a diet of the magical apricot. They first appeared in Britain during the reign of Henry VIII. Fresh apricots are only available in season, but the extracted oil is sold in chemists and health shops. Both fresh and dried apricots contain vitamin A, considered to be *the* skin vitamin. The fruit can be used in masks and the seeds to make a facial scrub. The oil makes a luxurious body lotion, and is thought to help eradicate stretch marks.

Avocado

The tree is indigenous to Central America, and the avocado has long been used there as a moisturizing protection against the sun. The fruit has a very high oil content plus lecithin and vitamins A and B. Fresh imported fruits are available most of the year, and the oil can be bought from herbalists and health shops. The rich oil is ideal for moisturizers and face masks and hair conditioners.

Banana

The first bananas seen in England in 1633 came from Bermuda, and they were regarded as a very exotic fruit by the British public. Shipments were soon obtained from the Canary Islands just off Africa. Bananas grow on an enormous plant which has white flowers in summer. The fruit is rich in vitamin A and potassium, making it excellent for a face mask.

Beer

Hops have grown wild for centuries, but by the Middle Ages they were being cultivated to make beer. It is the cones of the vine-like plant that are collected before maturity and dried for use by brewers. The leaves and flowerheads have been used in the past to make a brown dye. Beer gives body and shine to the hair, so is often used in shampoos and conditioners. Hops have been used for centuries as a filling for pillows to help insomniacs.

Blackberry

This is the commonest wild fruit in England, and has been eaten since earliest times. The familiar name bramble derives from the Anglo Saxon *bremel* meaning prickly. Blackberry is a hardy perennial with white flowers in summer followed by soft black fruits in early autumn. Many of our ancestors have pricked themselves on the thorns of this plant while blackberrying, and then used the crushed leaves to check the bleeding. Creeping under a bramble bush was thought to be a charm against boils and blackheads!

The fruit contains organic acids, pectin and albumen. The leaves contain a lot of tannin. Use the former as a face mask and the latter in astringents and lotions to refine the pores.

Bran

Bran is the coarse outer fibre on the wheat grain, and contains protein, riboflavin, thiamine and pantothenic acid. It is sold in

Blackberries grow in abundance in the wild, and the fruits are rich in organic acids. A poultice of crushed blackberries makes a good face mask to clear an oily complexion, and the leaves have a tightening action on the pores when used in skin tonics.

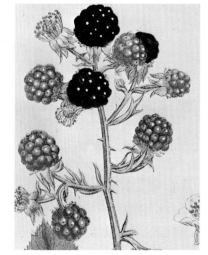

packets at most supermarkets, grocers and health food shops.

Its gritty particles make it a perfect addition to grainy facial and body scrubs, and it can be made into a soap for greasy skins.

Buttermilk

Buttermilk is a by-product of butter making, and resembles a watery milk. It contains the same nutrients as milk, such as calcium and protein, but is less fatty than whole milk for cosmetic purposes. Buttermilk makes an excellent cleanser when combined with other ingredients, and has a natural bleaching action to fade freckles. It can also be used to cool sunburnt skin.

Carrot

The carrot was well known to the ancients, and has been in constant use around the world. It was introduced to Britain by the Flemings in the reign of Elizabeth I, and in the reign of James I fashionable ladies took to wearing the feathery leaves in their head-dresses. The vegetable is available throughout the year.

Rich in vitamin A and B, carrot juice is a welcome additive to facial masks, skin milks and cleansers. A poultice of freshly grated carrot can relieve burns and inflammations.

Cinnamon

Cinnamon spice comes from the dried inner bark of the cinnamon tree, and it has a highly aromatic taste. When distilled it gives a delicious oil that contains an antiseptic. The ground bark is available from most delicatessens, while the essential oil can be obtained from herbalists.

Cinnamon has traditionally been chewed as a breath freshener, and the oil makes a luxurious and exotic body rub.

Cloves

Cloves are the dried buds of a small evergreen tree native to the Far East. The spice was introduced into Europe in the 4th century. They contain a large amount of essential oil which is antiseptic and much used in medicine. Cloves can be bought whole or ground from grocers. The oil is available from chemists and herbalists. Cloves make aromatic mouthwashes and breath fresheners, and a spicy oriental cologne.

Coconut

Coconut oil is extracted from the inner white flesh of the large nut. The tree is native to Malaysia. The oil can be bought from chemists, and is a rich, fine moisturizer. It can be used in hair conditioners, eye creams, lip salves, suntanning creams and hand creams.

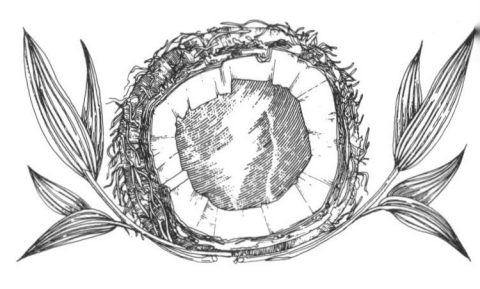

Cucumber

This most useful of beauty vegetables is native to the East Indies and has been used extensively since ancient times. It was first cultivated in England in the mid-17th century. It has the same acid-alkaline balance as the skin so cucumber is highly soothing, cooling and healing and can be used in toners, cleansers, face masks and is particularly useful in the treatment of painful sunburn.

Eggs

Eggs are rich in protein, iron and vitamins, and are one of the most versatile ingredients in beauty preparations. The egg white is highly astringent and is often used in face masks and hair setting lotions. The yolk makes a rich mask for dry skin and the whole egg is very beneficial when used as a hair conditioner.

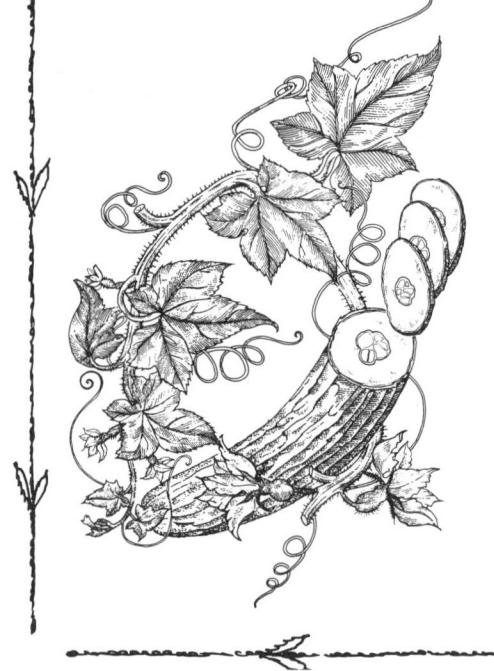

Grapefruit

The grapefruit gets its name from its habit of growing in clusters like grapes. It was recognized as a species in 1830 when it was thought to be a hybrid between a pomelo and an orange. The grapefruit is highly refreshing when used in skin toners, colognes, face masks and hair rinses. The rind can be used as a skin softener.

Honey

Honey is an ancient beauty aid and natural sweetener, derived from the nectar collected by bees. It is full of vitamins and minerals, and is an excellent moisturizer and healer of the skin. It also works well to bind other ingredients in cosmetics. Use it in soaps, face and body creams, masks and hand lotions.

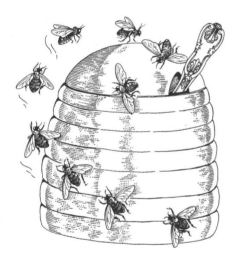

Lemon

The Arabs introduced the lemon to Spain and it has since spread to all parts of Europe. The fruits come from the lemon tree which is renowned for its beauty and its fragrant pink and white flowers. Because of its high vitamin C content, sailors have used it for years as protection against scurvy. Lemon juice neutralizes bacteria and when placed on oysters kills 90 per cent of their bacteria in 5 minutes.

If it is used after washing with soap, lemon juice restores the acid balance to the skin, and is highly astringent in toners, face masks, cleansing creams and lotions. A lemon rinse for fair hair leaves it clean and shining, and the bleaching action of lemon can be used on the hair, nails and on the skin to lighten freckles.

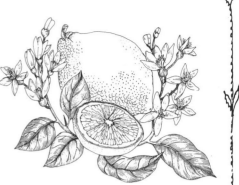

Lettuce

Lettuces were grown by the ancient Romans and Greeks – Cos lettuce comes from the Greek island of the same name. This vegetable has been grown in Britain since the Middle Ages. It is easily grown from seeds, or bought cheaply from greengrocers. Lettuces are rich in minerals: iodine, phosphorus, iron, copper, cobalt, zinc, calcium, manganese and potassium. They are an excellent additive to soaps, cleansers, toners and sunburn lotions.

Mayonnaise

This salad dressing contains eggs, oil and vinegar making it a complete cosmetic on its own! The egg has lecithin and protein, the vinegar restores the acid balance to the skin, and the oil is softening and moisturizing. Use it in face masks, cleansing creams and hair conditioners. To make 150ml (¼ pt) mayonnaise you will need:

150ml (¼ pt) oil
1 egg yolk
2 teaspoons vinegar
1 teaspoon boiling water

Put the oil in a jug, and put the egg yolk and half the vinegar into a bowl. Mix them together to blend. Whisk in half the oil, a few drops at a time, until the mayonnaise begins to thicken. Whisk in the remainder of the vinegar which will thin the mayonnaise a little, then hold the jug well above the bowl and pour the remaining oil on to the mayonnaise in a thin stream, whisking all the time until it thickens. Whisk in the boiling water to make a lighter consistency. This creamy mayonnaise will keep for a period of about three weeks, if kept continually in the fridge.

Melon

Cantaloups, honeydew, water and ogen melons are all rich in vitamins B and C. The first melons were cultivated in Africa by the Egyptians, and in later centuries they were produced in France. They make an excellent addition to face masks and cleansers and have a pleasant cooling effect.

Mustard

Both black and white mustard are wild herbs cultivated for their seeds and both have bright yellow flowers. When ground, the seeds form a pungent powder, and this has been used medicinally since ancient times. Hot water poured on the bruised seeds makes a stimulating footbath the steam from which can help dispel a cold, and a mustard bath also helps to tone up the circulation.

Oats

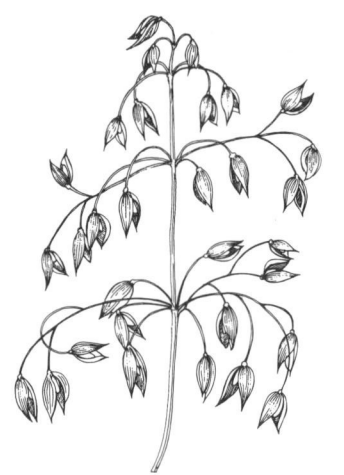

Oats grew wild throughout Europe from ancient times, but were not cultivated in Britain until the Iron Age. Romans believed them to be associated with the devil, and magicians used them in black magic. But doctors recommended their use in poultices to relieve inflammations, and the Scots adopted them as a staple of their diet. Oats are rich in protein, potassium, iron and magnesium. In the form of oatmeal they make an excellent beauty treatment as it helps to remove ingrained grime from the pores. It is particularly good to add to masks, scrubs, soaps and different types of cleansers.

Olive

The tree is mentioned in the Scriptures as a symbol of goodness, purity and happiness. Holding out an olive branch has long been used as an expression of peace. The oil, as well as its culinary use, was burnt in the temple lamps, while the victor of the Olympic Games was crowned with its leaves. The fine oil is often used nowadays as an additive to suntan lotions, it helps to feed very brittle nails and makes an excellent, rich hair conditioner.

Orange

Oranges originally came from China and one species, the mandarin, took its name from the vibrant robes of the noblemen. Oranges arrived in Europe brought by Arab traders. They regarded them as an emblem of happy marriage, and to this day brides wear orange blossom in their head-dresses. The Greeks still spray newlyweds with orangeflower water for luck. Oranges have always been regarded as a sign of opulence, and the Medici family took them as their own family symbol.

The fruit is full of vitamins A, B and C and phosphorus. Orange oil and flower water are frequent additions to skin fresheners, cleansers, moisturizers and colognes. The dried rind is an excellent addition to facial scrubs.

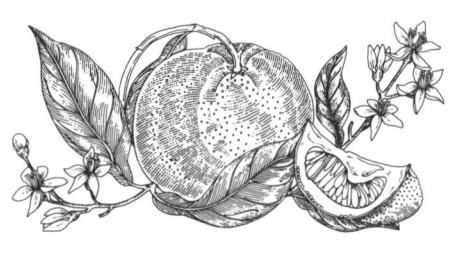

Orris

The root of the orris has long been used in perfumes, to clean clothing and as a tooth powder. Today the dried root makes an excellent dry shampoo.

Peach

The peach was brought to Europe by the Romans. They called it 'The Persian Apple' but it actually originated in China. The peach has the same place in Eastern mythology that the apple holds in the West. It was believed that the Gods ate peaches from a special tree, and this enabled them to live forever.

The oil extracted from the kernels has a lovely perfume and it can be bought from chemists. It is a rich addition to hair conditioners and moisturizers. The whole fruit can be used in face masks and cleansing lotions and creams.

Potato

The potato was introduced to Europe in the 16th century, brought by the Spaniards from the Andes. Sir Walter Raleigh was the first to plant the potato on his estate in Britain. At first they were considered a great delicacy, but soon became a staple of the diet. Potatoes are high in vitamins C and B, potassium and phosphorus. The raw grated potato is an excellent reliever of sunburn, and it can be used as a cleanser.

Safflower

The safflower plant is widely grown in India, China and Egypt, and is valued for its oil and the red dye obtained from the flowers. This is mixed with finely powdered talc to make rouge. The oil is extensively used in cooking, and is fine enough for use in moisturizers, cleansers and body oils.

Sesame

Sesame has been cultivated in the East for thousands of years. The seeds are eaten whole or ground into a paste called tahini. The oil from the seeds makes an excellent suntanning oil, and it is a good addition to hand and body lotions.

Rhubarb

Rhubarb is thought to have originated in Siberia. It is a hardy perennial which is grown for its thick red stems which have a sharp juice. The huge leaves are very poisonous. The roots of the plant release a yellow dye which gives hair a golden shine.

Strawberry

The first strawberries that grew wild in ancient Britain were tiny and dry. Early settlers in Virginia found sweet strawberries and brought them to England. Cross-breeding different strains has produced the large sweet fruits of today. Strawberries contain iron, organic acids and pectin. They have an astringent action on the skin making them an excellent addition to face masks, skin toners and cleansing milks.

Tomato

The tomato was originally known as the Love Apple, and arrived in Italy brought by the Spaniards in the 16th century. It has an astringent action and can be used as a face mask, a skin tonic and a cleanser.

Vinegar

The name derives from the French *vinaigre* meaning sour wine. Vinegars have been used for centuries to help the skin and hair. Most fruits become vinegar when fermented. Cider vinegar from apples is particularly beneficial cosmetically. Use it in face washes, hair rinses, and anti-dandruff lotions.

Wheatgerm

Wheatgerm is the wheat embryo contained in the heart of each grain. It is removed during the milling process and is rich in vitamins A, B and E, as well as copper, magnesium, phosphorus and calcium. You can buy dried wheatgerm from health shops, and wheatgerm oil from chemists.

Use dried wheatgerm in facial scrubs and masks. The oil is wonderfully fine in moisturizers, anti-wrinkle creams and eye creams.

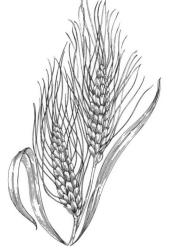

Yoghurt

Yoghurt is a milk product with a sour taste. An internal and external beauty aid, many bacteria are killed off by the acid it contains.

To make your own: You will need a thermometer and a wide-mouthed vacuum flask. Heat 600ml (1 pt) of skimmed UHT milk to 43°C (110°F). Stir in 2 tablespoons of dried skimmed milk and 1 tablespoon of live yoghurt. (All yoghurt is live unless it has been pasteurized). Transfer to a flask and leave for 4 to 5 hours in a warm place. The yoghurt will last about the same time as bought yoghurt (normally a week) if kept in the fridge.

Yoghurt is very beneficial to the skin and hair and can be included in many natural products. Use it in face masks, scrubs, cleansers and hair conditioners.

An A to Z of essential oils

The essential oils of plants and flowers are the vital fluids that exist in minute quantities. There are over 200 essential oils in existence, and about 30 of these are used by aromatherapists to cure a wide range of health and beauty problems. They are either massaged into the affected area or inhaled by the nose, from where they are believed to take a direct route to the brain and central nervous system. Therapists claim that just the fragrance of a certain flower can calm nerves and soothe aches and pains, while the scented oil can penetrate the skin's pores and permeate the bloodstream to cure inner ailments. Whether you believe this or not it is true that essential oils have antiseptic qualities, and they certainly delight the senses when added to baths and cosmetics.

Flowers and plants give up their vital essences sparingly. It takes 1 kilo of rose petals to produce one small bottle of rose oil, and 3000 lemons to make up 1 kilo of lemon oil. Complicated distillation processes are necessary, making the oils quite expensive. The oils are available to buy from herbalist shops (see page 119).

Essential oils added to cosmetics give them both fragrance and extra therapeutic qualities. Choose three or four basic essences to start with, then build up your collection from there. A good selection would be geranium, lavender, sandalwood and lemon verbena, giving a variety of differing scents. Or choose them according to your skin type. Dry skins will benefit from orange blossom, geranium, camomile and sandalwood, while oily skins will enjoy bergamot, juniper and cedarwood.

To make oils go further make flower waters, see the recipe on page 23.

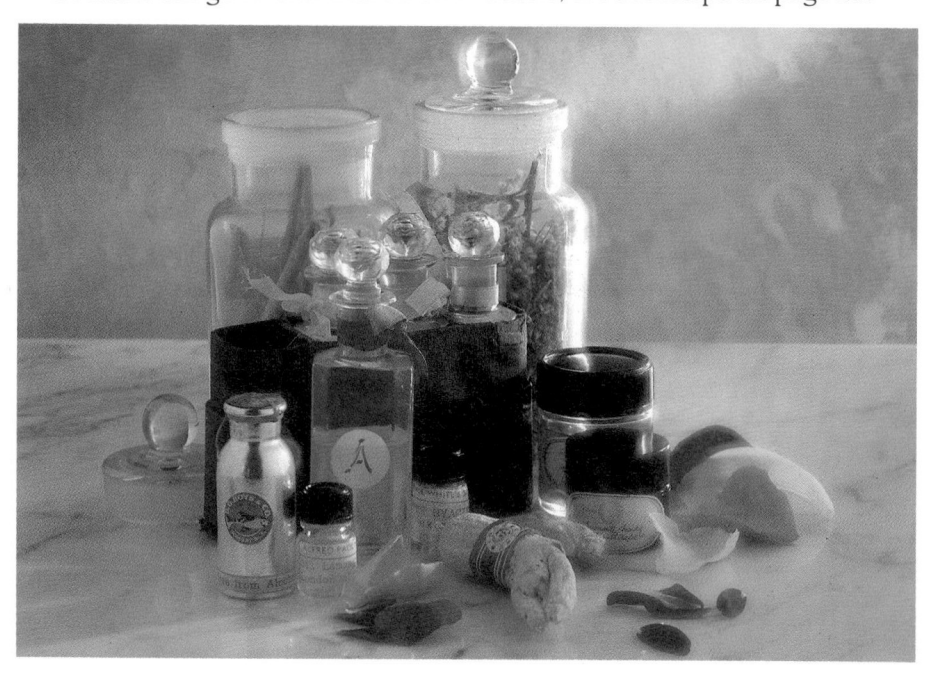

The essential oils of plants and flowers are the actual unadultered oils extracted from the plants in minute quantities. These true essential oils are ideal for adding perfume to natural cosmetics and they are also used in aromatherapy. They are expensive to buy, but cheaper versions can be bought in which a small amount of the essential oil has been diluted in sweet almond oil.

Angelica oil

A pale oil from the roots of the angelica herb, it smells musky and is often used in perfumes.

Bay oil

A yellow oil also known as Mycria oil used in perfumes.

Bergamot oil

Distilled from the peel of the bergamot fruit, it has an orangey smell and is added to perfumes and tanning lotions.

Camomile oil

A pale blue oil distilled from the camomile herb. Its light flowery scent makes it an excellent addition to face creams, especially ones for dry skin.

Cedarwood oil

A pale yellow, woody fragrance excellent in bath preparations.

Cinnamon oil

A yellow oil with a woody aroma, added to perfumes and bath preparations.

Clove oil

A pale yellow oil that is very stimulating. A renowned antiseptic and painkiller, it is frequently used to relieve the persistent pain of toothache.

Geranium oil

Also known as rose geranium oil it is a pale yellowish-green with a sweet fragrance. Particularly beneficial to ageing skin.

Jasmine oil

A light yellow oil distilled from the flowers, it has a sweet, exotic fragrance often added to perfumes. A few drops in the bath water soothes nervous tension.

Lavender oil

A pale yellowish-green oil with a sweet 'English garden' fragrance. Good for dry and irritated skins, and soothing in bath water.

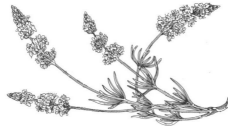

Lemon Verbena oil

A pale yellow oil distilled from the leaves of the verbena shrub with a sweet lemony scent. Ideal for oily skins.

Orange blossom oil

A clear oil with a sweet smell which is good for dry skins, and the scent is considered an effective anti-depressant when added to the bath.

Peppermint oil

A clear oil with a fresh cool scent, it clears congested sinuses and freshens the mouth in dental preparations.

Rose oil

One of the most precious of flower oils, its classic fragrance has enhanced perfumes and cosmetics for thousands of years. Distilled from red roses, it is very costly which puts it a little out of reach.

Sandalwood oil

Extracted from the wood of an evergreen tree native to India. Its exotic woody aroma makes it a favourite bath additive.

Ylang ylang oil

Distilled from the flowers of the *Cananga odorata* tree, native to Java. A sweet flowery oil often used in perfumes.

Peppermint oil, derived from the peppermint plant, is an inexpensive oil with a cool, invigorating fragrance. When inhaled it helps to relieve cold symptoms and a tiny drop rubbed over the teeth helps to freshen the breath.

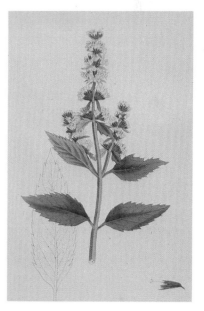

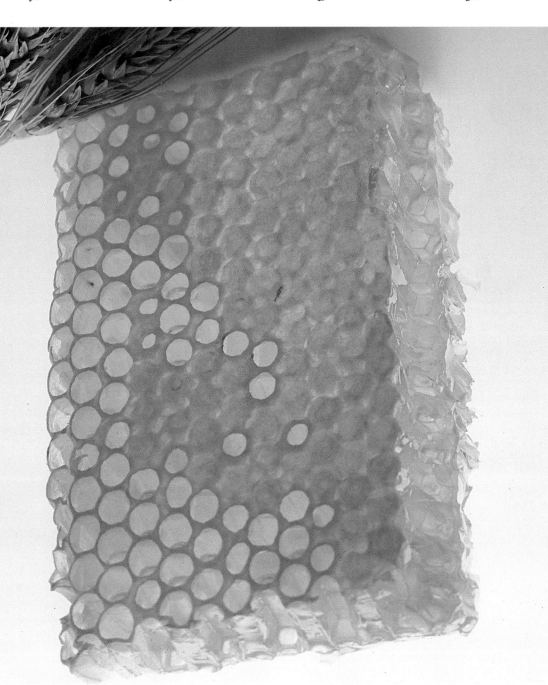

An A to Z of useful cosmetic ingredients

To make your cosmetics you will need various oils, waxes, resins and emulsifiers all of which are available or can be ordered from a major chemist. They are all listed here with their uses, along with some other useful ingredients.

Beeswax is used as a base for many face and body creams. It is the yellow wax that bees secrete when making the cells in honeycombs.

Alcohol

A pure alcohol of some kind is needed in cosmetics such as astringents, hair lotions and colognes for its antiseptic, drying and preserving properties. In a cologne, the alcohol lifts and diffuses a small amount of essential flower oil. In an astringent it dissolves excess facial oil and tightens the pores. Vodka is the perfect alcohol for cosmetic purposes as it is pure and made from grain. It is available from off licences and other normal retail outlets. Ethanol or industrial alcohol can be substituted and are available, on request, from most major branches of chemists.

Alum

Alum is a fine white crystalline powder made from aluminium and potassium salts. The granules are water soluble and have astringent properties. When made up into a solution they can be used in skin toner recipes.

Arrowroot

Arrowroot is a powdered starch extracted from the roots of a plant of the same name. It is used as a thickening agent in toothpastes and is also a good ingredient to use in dry shampoos.

Beeswax

Beeswax is a yellow wax secreted by bees to make the cells in honeycombs. To refine it to make white beeswax it is bleached and treated with acids. Chemists tend to sell it only in large quantities, so try to share with a friend. Beeswax acts as an emulsifying agent for oil and water, and has a high melting point making it ideal for face creams.

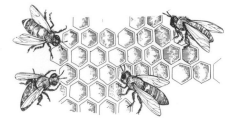

Benzoin

Benzoin is an aromatic resin from the Styrax tree, also known as gum benjamin. It has been used since ancient times in perfume and incense. Tincture of benzoin is the liquid from the gum, and can be added to creams and toners for its antiseptic and preserving qualities. Benzoic acid is the acid from the resin, and is used as a preservative.

Bicarbonate of soda

This is an acid salt of carbonic acid used in baking-powder and useful for cleaning the teeth.

Borax

A mineral found on alkaline lake shores, its transparent crystals have cleansing and astringent properties, and it acts as an emulsifier when added to oil and water to make face creams. Because of its detergent properties it is also added to soaps, cleansers, bath mixtures and hair shampoos.

Brewer's yeast

This yeast gets its name from the fact that it is used widely in the brewing industry. Yeasts contain minute fungi inducing fermentation, they are also rich in vitamins, minerals and proteins. Sold as a fine powder, brewer's yeast can be incorporated in a deep-cleansing face mask which is suitable for oily skins.

Calomine lotion

This is a lotion containing zinc carbonate. Its alkalinity makes it very soothing when applied to sunburnt skin and irritations.

Camphor

A solid essential oil from a species of cinnamon tree. It can be obtained as oil or spirit and is highly aromatic and stimulating to the skin. Added to a massage cream it improves the circulation and gives a warming sensation to aching muscles.

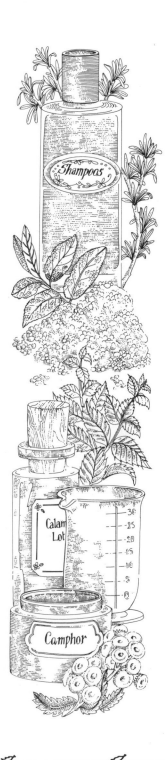

Castile soap

A pure white soap made from olive oil and caustic soda, with no added perfume, is known as Castile soap after the Spanish original. Use it grated to make your own soaps, shampoos and bath gels.

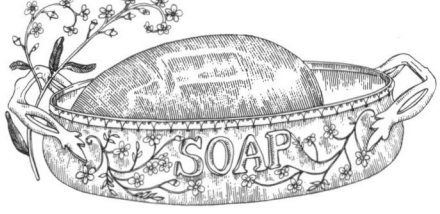

Castor oil

Castor oil is obtained from the seeds of the African plant, *Ricinus communis*. A smooth rich oil, it is used in commercial lipsticks and soaps, and is excellent as a hair and nail conditioner, in lip salves and as a body oil.

Cocoa butter

This is a fat obtained from the cocoa-bean which makes a rich oily addition to body creams.

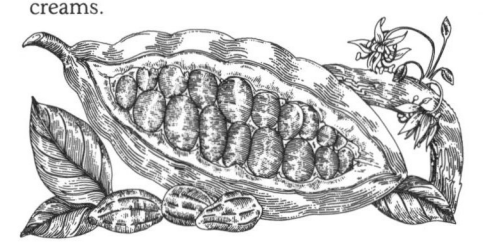

Coconut oil

An oil extracted from the white meat of the nut, it is an excellent addition to face and body creams, and hair conditioners.

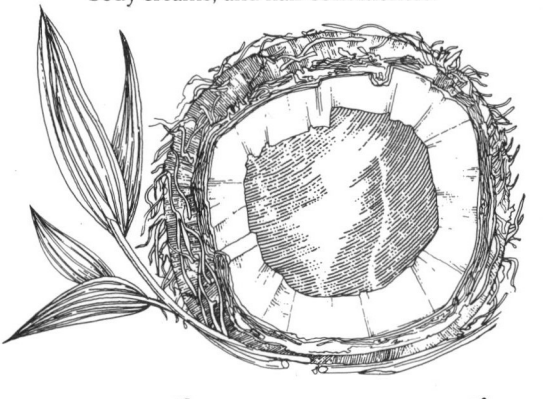

Emulsifying wax

As the name explains, this is wax which is very efficient at emulsifying oil and water in creams. It is made from ceto stearyl alcohol and lauryl sulphate.

Fuller's earth

A fuller was a person who finished cloth, and fuller's earth is an earthy hydrous aluminium silicate used to absorb grease and clean wool. This absorbent clay is rich in minerals, and can be used in cleansing face masks for its excellent drawing and stimulating properties.

Gelatine

This is a colourless, odourless and tasteless glue prepared from bones and hides, and a rich source of protein. It can be used as a setting lotion and as a base in nail hardening lotions.

Glycerine

This is an odourless and colourless liquid which is soluble in water. It is a by-product of soap making. It is a humectant, which means it attracts and holds water. Because of its lubricating qualities it is often included in hand and body lotions, liquid soaps and bath gels, toners, fresheners and hair lotions.

Gum resins

A gum resin, such as gum tragacanth, is a natural resin obtained from trees. It is used as a thickening emulsifier in creams, toothpastes and setting lotions.

Kaolin

This is a china clay sold as a fine white powder which has binding and drawing powers making it ideal for face masks.

Kelp

Kelp is a seaweed rich in minerals which makes it an excellent additive to face masks.

Lanolin

Lanolin is the sebum or oil that is extracted from sheep's wool. It is widely used in commercial moisturizers and body lotions. It is normally only sold in fairly large quantities, so try to share with a friend. There are two types of lanolin – anhydrous which is thick and tacky, and hydrous which has added water making it thinner. Unless otherwise specified, anhydrous lanolin is most frequently used in the recipes detailed.

Lecithin

This is a highly complex substance containing phosphorus found in egg yolk and soya beans, and animal proteins. Sold as a soft beige powder it is nourishing in masks and creams.

Myrrh

Myrrh in an aromatic, transparent gum exuded from the bark of the sweet cicely shrub. Since ancient times it has been valued for its antiseptic and preservative qualities, which is why it was used in the East for mumification. Sold as a tincture it is useful for adding shelf life to creams and lotions, and for making tooth powders and mouth washes.

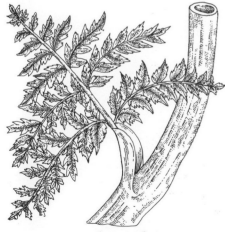

Oleic acid

A liquid prepared from oil which has emulsifying properties. A couple of drops added to a cream that is separating will soon bind it together.

Petroleum jelly

A mineral jelly widely used commercially in lip salves and hand and nail creams.

Salt

Sea salt can be used to clean the teeth and as an abrasive body rub to remove rough skin and improve the circulation.

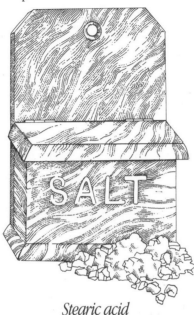

Stearic acid

A natural fatty acid added as an emulsifier to hand and body creams.

Sulphur

A mineral powder used in acne preparations to inhibit the flow of oil from the oil glands.

Witch hazel

A distillation of the bark of the witch-elm dissolved in alcohol, used in skin tonics for its astringent properties.

Zinc oxide

A white powder derived from the metallic element zinc, often used in paint pigments. It has mildly astringent and antiseptic qualities, and can be used as a dusting powder or in a soothing lotion.

Basic equipment and methods

The right equipment, set aside just for making your cosmetics, will make life simple, and help you to feel professional. This list is meant as a guideline, but it is not necessary to buy anything at all – you can improvise with utensils in your kitchen, but do clean thoroughly before and after use.

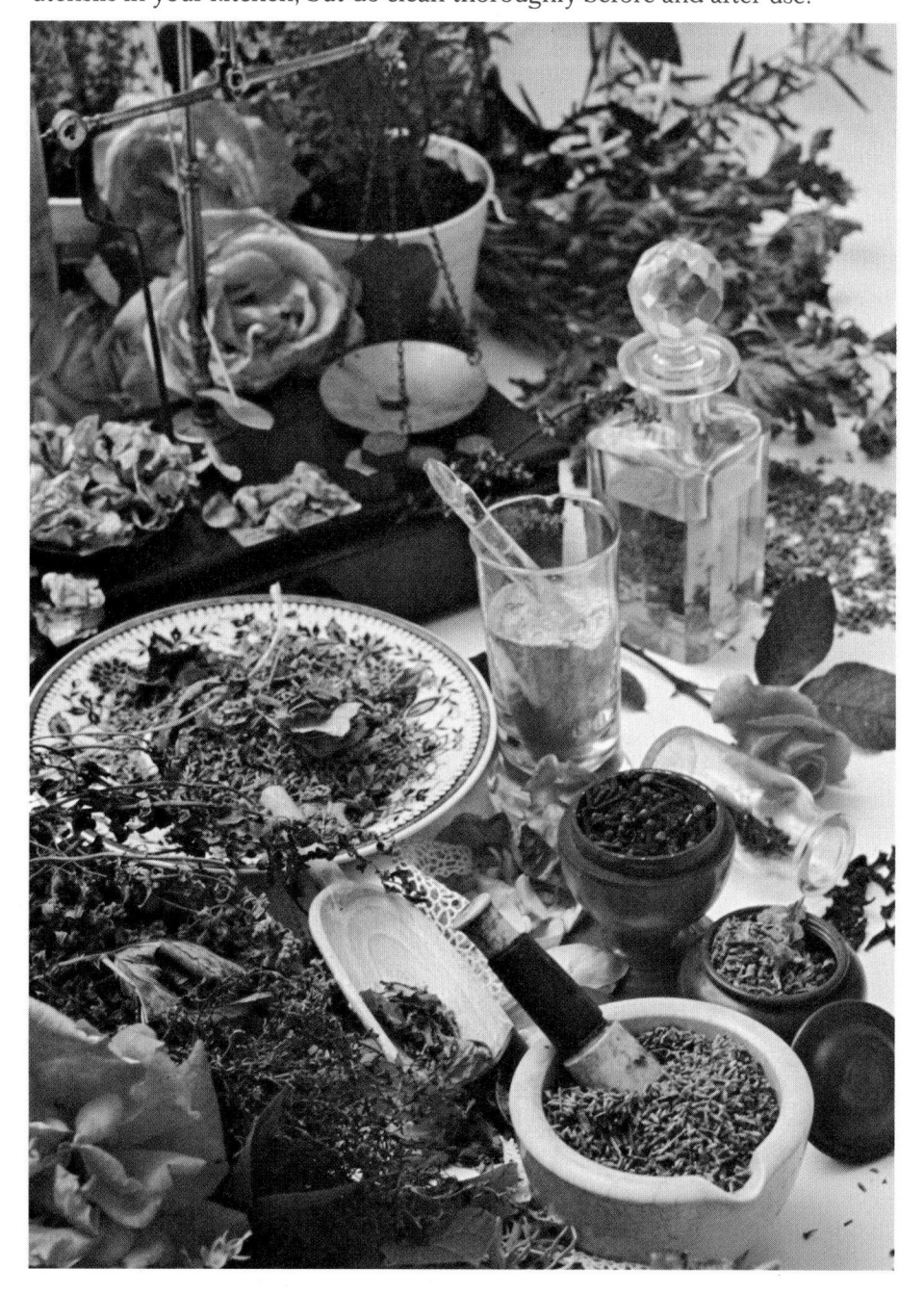

You can make your cosmetics using simple equipment that you probably already possess, but it helps to set aside a selection of spoons and containers just for your beauty products. Bottles that are used for other purposes should be sterilized well after use.

You will need the following items, or an improvised alternative:
An enamel-coated (not metal) double boiler (or a large saucepan or roasting tin in which to place heat-resistant glass, enamel or earthenware bowls).
Small scales
An electric or hand whisk
A pestle and mortar
A fine nylon sieve
A grater
Measuring jug(s)
Small funnels
Measuring spoons
Wooden spoons
An eye dropper
A plastic spatula
A liquidizer
Dark glass jars and bottles
Labels
Kitchen paper (For wiping utensils free of oil between use)

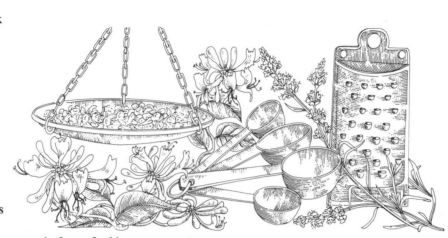

Bottling and labelling

You can buy dark glass bottles and pots from the chemist quite cheaply, or collect old medicine and cosmetic pots – wide-topped varieties are best, and make sure they have well-fitting lids. They must be dark glass because this protects the contents against deterioration from exposure to sunlight.

If you are re-using old bottles, it is important to wash and sterilize them thoroughly beforehand. Wash them in hot soapy water, then fill them half full with alcohol (an industrial variety from the chemist is cheaper than using vodka) and half with water, and leave to stand for 12 hours. Rinse in hot water and dry thoroughly.

It is very important to label each cosmetic as you go along, because after you have made several you are bound to forget the ingredients that went into each one. Write on the label with a ballpoint pen (inks and felt-tip pens tend to smudge) before you stick it onto the pot or bottle, and if you are artistic you could make a drawing of the herb or flower used. Spraying labels with artists' fixative helps to keep them from fading.

Keep your own recipe book

Just as our great-grandmothers and their ancestors before them used to write down their recipes in a book, it is a good idea for you to keep your own record so that you will always be able to refer back to those recipes which worked out well for your needs. You may well find that some combinations of oils and waxes suit your skin type better than others, and that certain herbs and flowers give you better results. Experiment with your own recipes

– the perfect cosmetics for you are not the same as for someone else. This is the beauty of natural cosmetics – you can make the ideal skin and hair care range designed exclusively for you.

Perfecting the methods

When you first start making your own cosmetics you may find you have to practise a few times to get the recipes right. This is particularly true when making creams and lotions containing oils, waxes and waters. Oil and water are notoriously unwilling to mix – think how easily they separate when mixed in a french dressing.

The right amount of emulsifier such as a wax or borax will encourage oil and water to *stay* mixed, but when adding a lot of water to a little oil to make a lotion, a great deal of energetic whisking will be needed at the crucial stage. If the ingredients have cooled down and separated, simply heat the mixture and start whisking again. If they still fail to bind, throw the lot away and start again.

It is important when you start out to keep to the measures exactly, 15g (½oz) more or less of any ingredient can make a lot of difference to the final

The balance of oils and waters used in your cosmetics determines their consistencies. As you get more practised at making your own creams you can alter the proportions of ingredients to suit you.

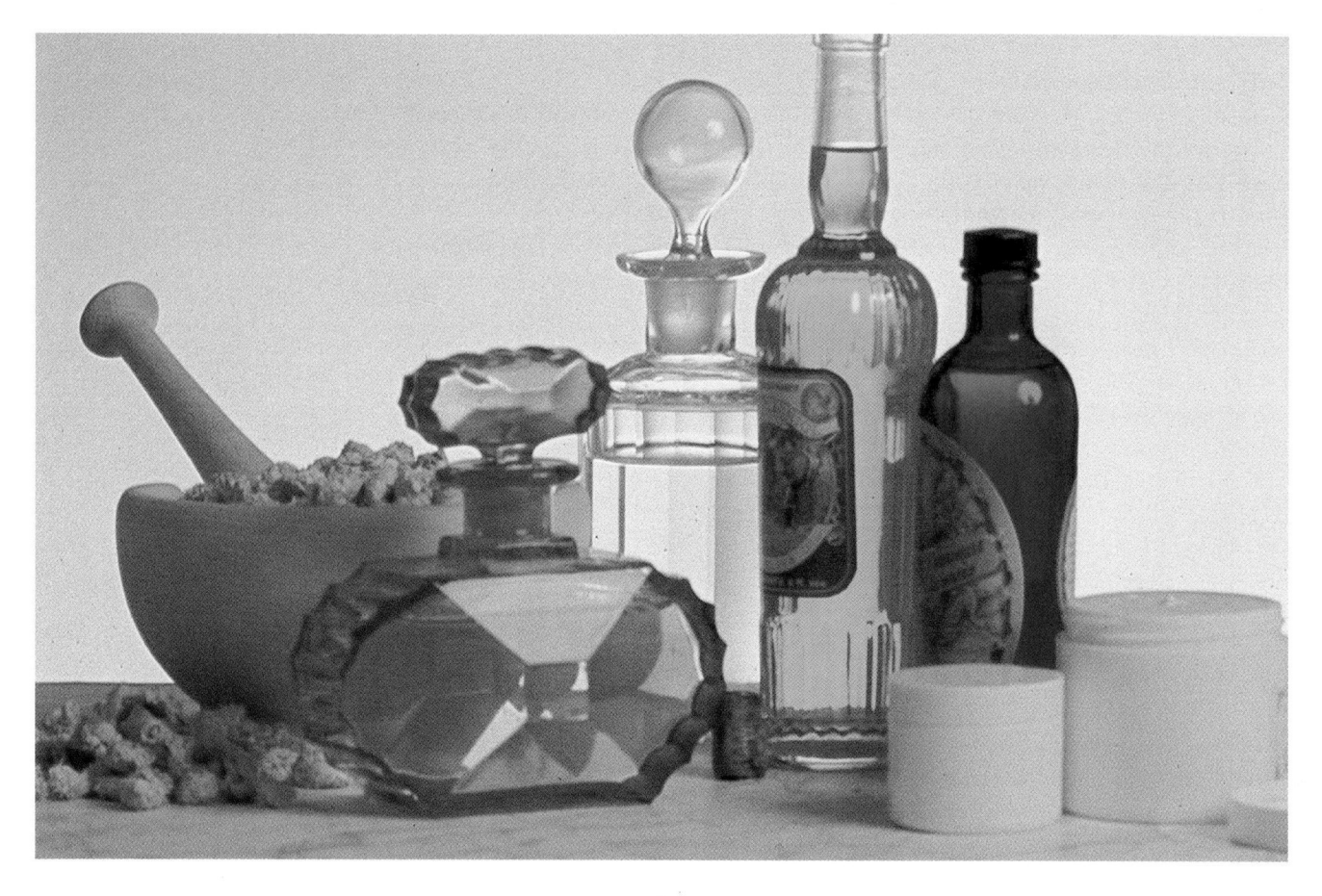

product. Later when you are familiar with the properties of each substance, you can change the balance to suit you. Keep trying until you get the consistency you like – adding more wax makes a cream stiffer, more oil will make it oilier, and more water will make it runnier and harder to bind.

A basic cream

The method for making a basic cream is very simple, and from this recipe all other varieties of creams are made. Four parts of oil (vegetable oil or a similar type) are heated with one part of wax. Two parts of water are heated separately, and then both the oil and wax mixture and the water are removed from the stove and stirred together until cool. Adding a pinch of borax to the heating water helps the emulsifying process. When the mixture is cool, a few drops of a flower or herb oil are added for perfume. And that is it – a light, white delicious face cream, perfect for cleansing or moisturizing. More oil will make a richer moisturizer, more water will make a more fluid cleansing lotion. More wax will make a harder moisturizer for lip salves.

When using herb or flower infusions instead of plain purified water in a cream, it is necessary to add some preservative to give shelf life. Tinctures of benzoin and myrrh are added for this purpose.

Allergy testing

The one drawback with natural ingredients is that just as many people are allergic to them as they are to the synthetic substitutes. So patch test a little of each one before you include it in your cosmetics. It is worth testing them on the area where the cosmetic will be applied – some people find their facial skin reacts to lanolin but it is perfectly acceptable on the hands and body.

Here are some common ingredients which can cause allergic reactions:
Almond oil
Camphor
Cocoa butter
Glycerine
Ivy
Lanolin
Nettles
Strawberries
Tincture of benzoin
Tincture of myrrh
Essential oils can also cause allergies, especially on the face. Some common ones are:
Bay
Bergamot
Geranium
Orange blossom
Peppermint

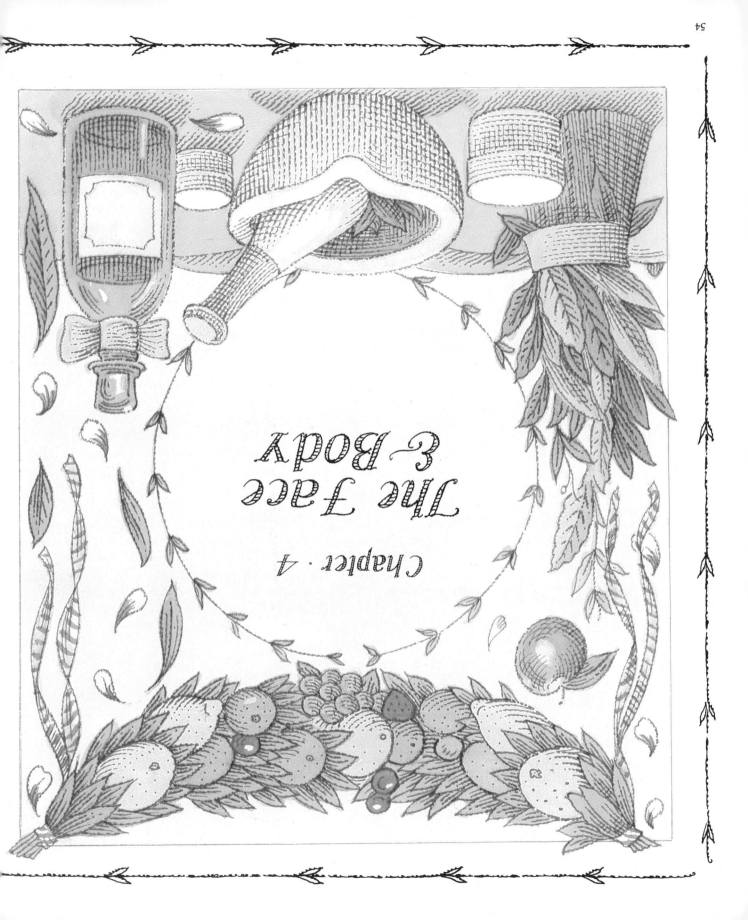

Chapter · 4

The Face
& Body

The face

A good skin is the foundation of beauty. A perfect healthy skin is smooth and supple to the touch, evenly coloured with a delicate blush, and glows with a soft translucence. If your facial skin looks this good without encouragement you are extremely lucky, because most women have to take considerable care to keep their skins in peak condition.

If your skin looks out of sorts, it will make you feel unhappy, too. Both your inner health and outer environmental conditions affect the appearance of your skin, and blemishes, dry flaky patches, oily areas and blocked pores are far more common than a flawless complexion.

Understanding the basic structure and functions of your skin will help you correct the balance when something goes wrong. Because only then can you choose the right skin care programme to restore your skin to health.

The cosmetic industry often makes sweeping claims for its products – creams and lotions are said to 'feed' growing skin cells, restore elasticity to ageing skin, close pores and remove blemishes. Many of these claims are unscientific or just not true. Know how your skin works, and not only can you analyze these claims, you can make superior products that will be better suited to your own personal needs.

The skin's functions

Although your skin is only a few millimetres thick, it is a highly complex and hard-working organ just like your heart, lungs or liver. It protects your internal tissues from dehydration and damage, acts as a barrier to stop bacteria getting into the body, and lets out excess water, minerals and salts through sweat.

Your skin helps to regulate your body temperature. To cool you down in hot weather, or after strenuous exercise, the blood vessels near the skin's surface dilate, so that warm blood can be carried close to the outside air to be cooled down. This is why you flush red when hot. Sweat cools down the body too. It is produced all over the skin in a fine layer of moisture which evaporates off into the air. On a cold day the body needs to conserve warmth, so these tiny blood vessels contract and divert the blood inwards, leaving the skin looking pale.

If you cut your skin it is remarkably self-healing. The average skin is damaged many hundreds of times in a lifetime, but restores itself, through the body's efficient healing processes, to a smooth continuous layer in a matter of days.

Nerve endings in the skin provide a constant early warning system against danger. Some nerves are designed to pick up pain, others touch, and still others hot and cold sensations.

No wonder such a complex structure as your skin can occasionally seem temperamental. But do not blame the surface skin cells that you can see if

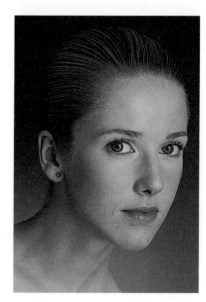

A healthy skin should be smooth, supple and blemish-free, and reflect both your inner health, your daily diet and the amount of care you take of your complexion.

your skin does not look as good as it should. These cells are dead, and it is deeper down in the skin's inner layers that troubles begin.

The skin's layers

To understand your skin's construction from the inside out, it is worth looking at the body in the same way. Inside your body are your internal organs, then your skeleton, then muscles, then a layer of fat, then two layers of skin: the dermis and the epidermis. If the layer of fat is thick and uneven it will effect the appearance of the skin by stretching and dimpling it. If this layer of fat is rapidly reduced by dieting, the skin will remain stretched but appear loose.

The dermis

The skin's thicker inner layer is the dermis, and this is where the glands that produce sweat and oil are located. Taking up more space are nerve endings and hair follicles, and all the blood vessels necessary to nourish the skin by carrying proteins, fats, vitamins and minerals to the growing cells, and also taking away waste matter. These tiny blood vessels give the skin its rosy colour. If some of them become permanently dilated through losing their ability to contract again they become visible as 'thread' veins.

The glands that produce oil are known as the sebaceous glands, and they have a vital role to play in the appearance of your skin. These glands are attached to the sides of each hair follicle, and the oil (called sebum) that they produce forms a coating on the emerging hairs that then spreads out as a thin film over the surface of the skin. The point of this oil is to help the skin cells on the surface retain water, and so keep their smooth appearance. The oil is also slightly acidic, defending the skin against bacteria.

The hair follicles on your scalp produce hairs that grow thick and long, but over the face and body the hairs are fine or non-existent – unlike the days when we were covered all over with hair for protection! These hair follicle exits are visible on the skin as pores. If the supply of oil coming out of these pores is too generous, the skin will appear greasy, and sebum will block up the pores forming spots. If the supply of sebum is too meagre, the skin will appear dry and flaky. The amount of oil the glands produce is governed by your hormones, and some areas like the forehead, cheeks, chin and upper back have extra large glands.

Collagen and elastin

The dermis, through which all these glands, hair follicles and blood vessels thread their way, is made up of fibrous connective tissue. Most of this is collagen, a strong protein also found in tendons, cartilage and bone. The rest is elastin, and these two proteins together give the skin its elasticity and strength. If you pinch your skin you will find it snaps back immediately into shape. But as the skin ages, the collagen and elastin fibres start hardening and shrinking, and so wrinkling begins.

A cross-section of a piece of skin, magnified many times, shows that it is divided into several layers. The outer layer, known as the epidermis contain no blood vessels or nerves – these are situated in the dermis below. This inner layer is made of strong connective tissue, and when this breaks down the skin starts to age. Under the dermis is a layer of fat which can affect the appearance of the skin by stretching and dimpling it, as in the case of people who are overweight.

Epidermis

Dermis

Collagen and elastin

Subcutaneous fat

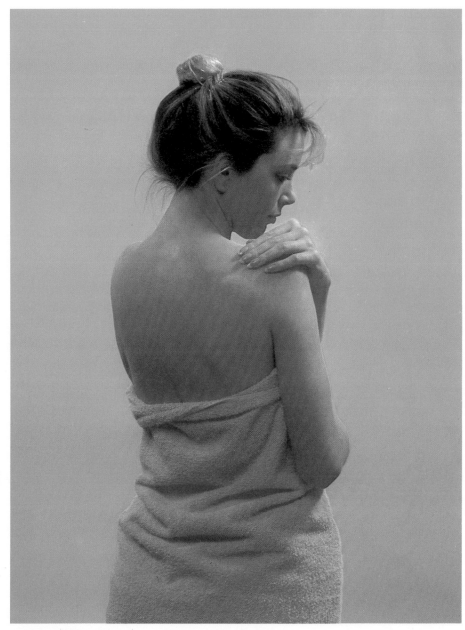

The epidermis

This is the skin's visible outer layer, and it is layered in turn. It is very thin and has no blood vessels or nerves, but is a powerhouse of activity. Deep in the epidermis, in the basal layer, new skin cells are formed. Dead cells are continuously flaking off the surface of the skin, so fresh supplies of cells from below are constantly in demand. In the basal layer, the new skin cells are fed by nutrients diffusing up from the dermis below. A new cell is created by one cell splitting in two – one half stays where it is and the other half, once completely formed, starts moving upwards to the skin surface, taking between two to four weeks to get there. It leaves the basal layer plump with moisture, but as it moves upwards it grows thinner and harder, secreting a tough, flexible protein called keratin as it goes. Once fully keratinized the cell is no longer alive.

Dead cells lie on the surface of the skin, tightly packed and flattened out to form a strong continuous, perfectly interlocked jigsaw. Although they are dead, there is enough water retained in each cell to preserve the softness and flexibility of the skin.

The keratin layer is the very outer layer of skin which is continuously being shed in microscopic fragments as new cells rise up and replace the old ones. This outer layer is also subjected to friction from your clothes, and every time you scratch yourself you are removing many more.

These surface cells will not fit smoothly together if they were poorly formed in the first place from under-nourished basal cells, and they will not look sleek and translucent if they cannot flake off easily and evenly because they are stuck together with oil and make-up that has not been carefully removed. Conversely over-strenuous cleansing with harsh soaps and astringents can remove too much oil and the water content of the cells, so that they become over-dried and curl up at the edges, giving the skin a cracked and flaky appearance.

Your skin colour

Whether you are dark or fair skinned depends on how many melanin cells you have deep in the epidermis. These cells produce a brown pigment which responds to sunlight and produces a suntan, to protect the skin against burning. Ultra violet light from the sun can get through the skin and damage the living cells in the basal layer. These rays can also penetrate the dermis and destroy collagen, so causing the skin to lose its elasticity. A suntan is really a sign of the skin protecting itself against damage as melanin cells go into production. There is no way you can alter your skin's ability to create melanin, so the fair-skinned should always approach sunbathing with caution.

Your facial skin type

Although all human skin has the same basic structure, the oil and water content varies a great deal from person to person. Dividing skin types into the categories of dry, oily, combination and sensitive enables you to decide on which side of normal your skin falls. A normal skin is smooth, soft and blemish free, needing the absolute minimum of outside care to keep it looking good.

Less fortunate people need to keep an eye on their skins from day to day, and treat them according to their changing needs. Do not assume that just because you have decided you have oily skin you can find one simple skin care regime and stick to it rigidly throughout the year. Oily skins can

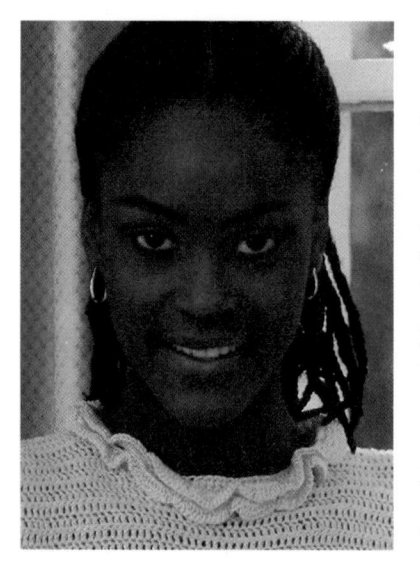

Differences in skin colour are due to different levels of melanin. Melanin granules are produced in the epidermis by cells called melanocytes. Sunlight speeds up the action of the melanocytes.

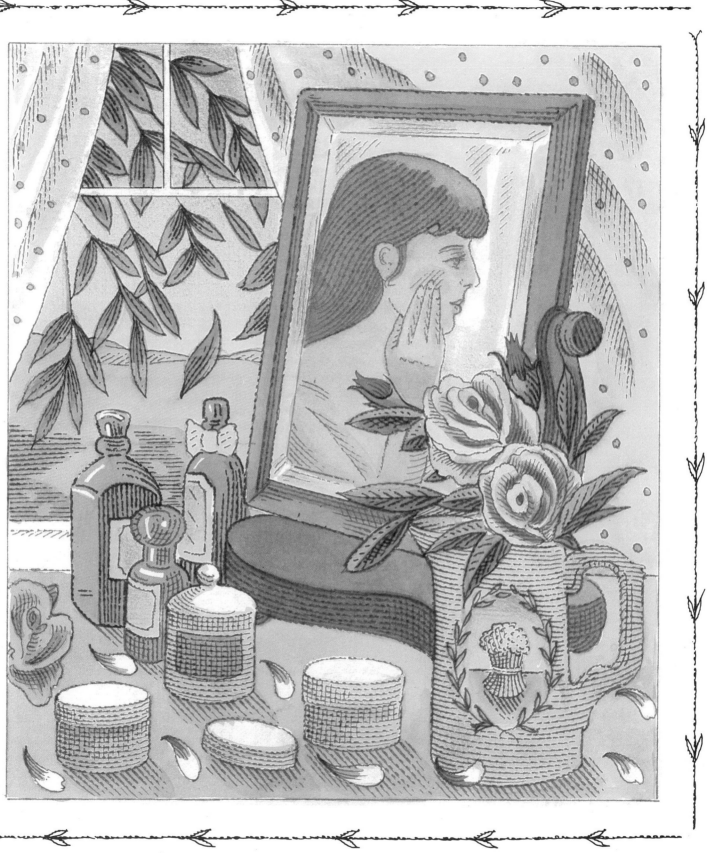

develop dry patches and dry skins can suddenly find they are getting oilier – it all depends on the weather and the changes in your health and lifestyle.

Skin secretions change as you get older, so it is important that skin care is kept up to date. Over-cleansing a dry skin could do it more damage than not cleansing it at all, while neglecting to remove stale oil from a greasy skin will soon lead to spots.

To discover the oil and water balance of your skin today, follow this simple test.

Remove all traces of make-up and wash your face with a mild unperfumed soap. Rinse well and pat dry, but do not use a toner or moisturizer. Now leave your skin to settle for two hours, then examine it in a strong light with a mirror.

Dry skin

A dry skin will look matt with no hint of shine, and it will feel tight. If it is very dry there may be patches of flaking and peeling skin, and wrinkles will look prominent as the thin epidermal layer has fallen into the underlying wrinkles in the dermis. (There are no wrinkles in the outer layer itself.) The pores will be invisible and tiny veins may show up around the nose and cheeks. Your skin will feel as if it is crying out for moisture to restore suppleness to its texture. All skins become drier as they get older, and more vulnerable to changes in outside temperatures. The plus factor in this skin type is that you are unlikely to get spots, and your pores will hardly be noticeable. But a very dry skin can become cracked enough for bacteria to penetrate through the outer keratin layer, leading to unsightly blemishes. You must treat your skin very gently using the mildest of cleansers, and moisturize lavishly whenever you feel the need.

Oily skin

An oily skin will look shiny all over, and feel supple. So much sebum may have risen to the surface on the forehead, nose and chin that the skin feels oily to the touch. The pores will be very noticeable, and many will be blocked with stale oil and dead skin cells. These blackheads occur where the exits of the hair follicles become narrowed, and the flow of oil to the surface becomes blocked so that it accumulates under the surface. These blackheads can only be removed by squeezing them out, but afterwards the pores can not be closed whatever you do to them. If the hair follicles are totally blocked, oil builds up under the surface and forms acne spots. These cannot be squeezed out unless they have a definite head. The only course of action is to leave them alone for the skin to disperse from the inside. Rupturing the skin can spread infection and lead to a scar, which will add to the coarsened appearance of a greasy skin.

This skin type needs constant care, but removing excess oil must be gently done or the glands will produce even more oil to compensate. Frequent washing with mild soap followed by the use of very mild antiseptics is your best course of action. Consoling facts are that your skin is

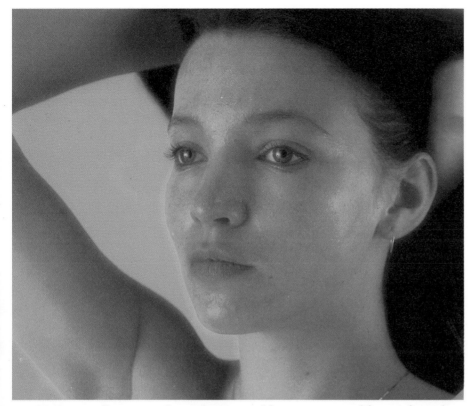

less likely to collapse into lower lying wrinkles as you get older, and it is less vulnerable to excesses of sun and wind.

Combination skin

This is by far the most common skin type, and is like owning the skins of two separate people. The centre panel of the face will show a shine like a oily skin, while the outside of the cheeks and around the eyes will stay tight and dry. To care for your skin moisturize the outer drier areas frequently, and cleanse the oily centre panel at the same time.

Sensitive skin

This type of skin usually belongs to blondes or redheads or anyone with very fair skin. It reacts to strong soaps and perfumed cosmetics by coming up in bumps and rashes, and quickly goes red and burns in the sun. People with sensitive skins often flush easily or come out in blotches after contact with chemical substances. You will always have to choose your cosmetics very carefully. Making your own skin care products is ideal for you because you can experiment with different ingredients to see which ones you are allergic to, then mix your creams to suit your sensitivity.

Keeping your skin in tip-top condition

Follow these simple guidelines and you will be doing everything possible to protect your skin's good health and appearance.

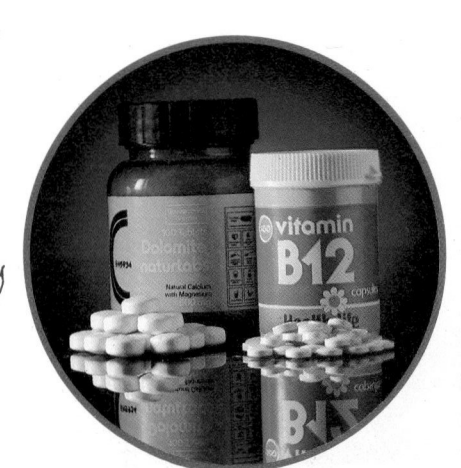

Vitamins are essential for the formation of healthy skin tissues. Vitamin supplements are only necessary if you do not eat a balanced diet, or when suffering from illness.

● **Watch your diet.** Unhealthy eating soon shows up in your skin, especially if there is a shortage of fresh fruit and vegetables. Your body needs vitamins – these are organic compounds found in commonplace foods – and there is no need to take vitamin supplements if your diet is well balanced.

Vitamin A is know as the skin vitamin and is often added to face creams. Ideally it should be added to your diet where it can work from the inside out. It is found in eggs, liver, milk, butter, cheese and dark coloured vegetables such as carrots and tomatoes. Too little of this vitamin causes dry skin and dry eyes, but it is the only vitamin that can poison you if you take too much, so never take a supplement.

Vitamin B complex is often thought of as the 'women's vitamin' as it has many important roles to play in the various systems of the body, and vitamin B6 is particularly renowned for its help for sufferers of pre-menstrual tension. Vitamin B includes B1 (thiamine), B2 (riboflavine), B6 (pyridoxin), B12, folic acid, pantothenic acid and biotin. These vitamins are found in cereals, milk, eggs, liver, meat and green vegetables.

Vitamin C is essential for healthy skin and is found in fresh fruit and vegetables. Without it wounds fail to heal properly and weakened blood vessels cause bleeding under the skin.

Vitamin D keeps the bones healthy and is necessary to help the body absorb calcium. It is found in fish, eggs and milk.

Vitamin E is found in wheatgerm oil, in many plant seeds and in leafy vegetables. Little is known of its actions – it is added to many face creams as it is believed to improve the texture of the skin.

Calcium is necessary for strong skin, nails and hair. It is found in cheese, milk, eggs, green vegetables, oranges, nuts, beans and carrots.

Vitamin B complex has many important functions in the body. It is found in the greatest quantities in cereals and grains, wholemeal bread, liver, potatoes, beer and green vegetables.

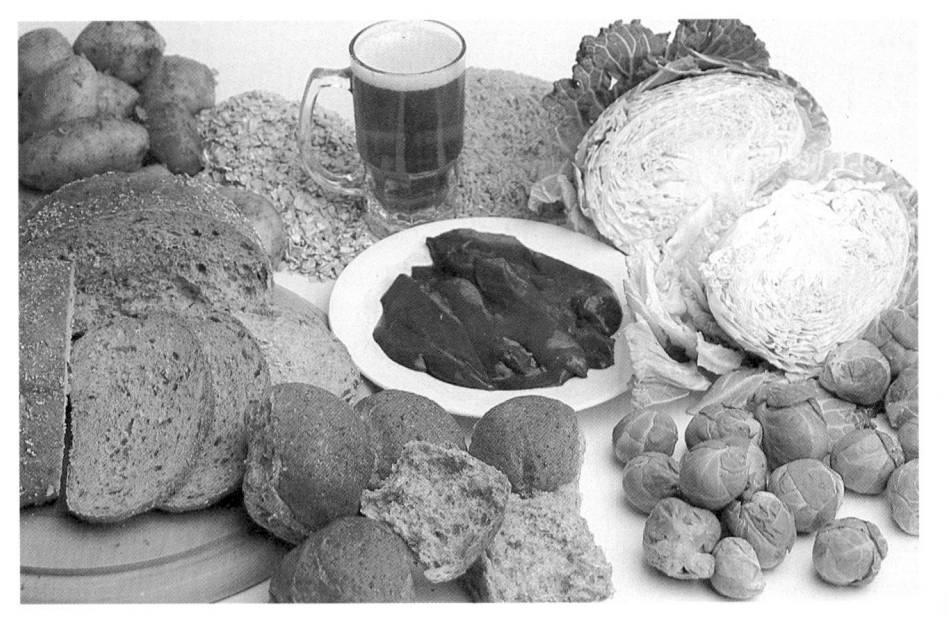

Iron is needed by the blood – a deficiency causes anaemia. It is found in meat, liver, kidney, eggs, green peas, spinach, watercress, cabbage, carrots and cereals.

Other substances needed in tiny amounts are potassium, magnesium, iodine, phosphorus, sulphur, copper, cobalt, manganese and zinc. The average diet provides enough of these to make supplements unnecessary.

● **Drink plenty of water** – at least two pints a day to flush out your system. Tea and coffee do not count, you should drink plain water, sparkling mineral water or unsweetened fruit juices.

● **Keep your skin protected** against over-exposure to sun and wind. If you feel unhealthy without a tan in summer, keep the sun off your face and hands by wearing a sunscreen cream. These areas have the most delicate skin and will age quickly if not protected. In cold weather apply a moisturizer frequently to avoid chapped, cracked skin.

● **Beware of the dangers** of central heating – the air in a room can become so dry that moisture is rapidly lifted from the skin. Keep the thermostat down as low as is comfortable, and keep small bowls of water as simple humidifiers by radiators.

● **Keep your skin clean** but do not dry it out with harsh products. Always use mild cleansers, but use them frequently if your skin feels grimy or oily. If your skin feels fine, leave it alone.

● **Do not wear** make-up all the time – your skin needs fresh air and make-up stops skin cells flaking off with ease, leading to a stale build-up on the skin surface.

● **Get plenty of outdoor exercise** to keep the circulation of the blood working well and the skin well fed.

● **Make sure you have enough sleep.** The hormones responsible for cell division and the renewal of skin tissues are most active while you sleep, so lack of sleep will lead to tired, lifeless-looking skin.

● **Keep alcohol to a minimum** – it dehydrates the whole body, including the skin.

● **Try to avoid** touching your face and picking at spots – this spreads bacteria and hinders natural recovery. Always treat blackheads carefully. Use tissues to cover the fingers when squeezing them, and dab a mild antiseptic afterwards.

● **Try to relax** – tension can make your skin oilier and screwing up the face speeds wrinkles. This is why you may get a spot before an important occasion – your nervous system causes your hormones to trigger increased oil production, and excess oil can get blocked in the pores.

Cleansing

Thorough cleansing is the most important part of skin care. Your skin is constantly collecting grime from the atmosphere which combines with the natural oil on the skin's surface, and if this dirt is not regularly cleaned away

Below and bottom: Massaging the skin helps to stimulate the blood circulation and eases away tension. Treat yourself to a facial massage at night when applying your moisturizer. Work from the chin up to the temples, using the backs of your fingers in a firm, stroking movement.

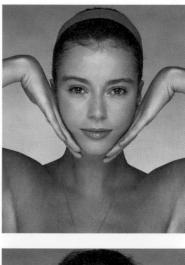

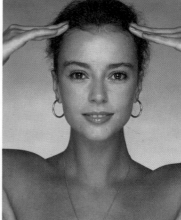

it can collect in the pores and lead to unsightly spots.

Everyone's skin is highly individual and needs a carefully thought out cleansing routine. The drier your skin, the more gentle your products need to be, while oily skins never feel really clean unless they have been washed in soap and water. Another factor to take into account is the way your skin changes from day to day according to your general health and even the weather.

All skin types need to be cleaned very gently in the morning and more thoroughly at night. Only very oily skins need to be cleaned more often than this, as excess cleaning will strip away too much oil leading to sensitive, irritated skin.

Whether you clean your face with soap and water or just with creams is a matter for personal preference, but all skins enjoy an occasional soapy wash. Soap is not as efficient as cream cleansers at removing make-up, as oil is needed to dissolve the waxes and pigments in cosmetics. The best solution for normal and oily skins is a cream cleanse followed by soap and water, and cream only cleansing for dry skins, with a once a week soap wash using the mildest of herbal soaps.

All about soap

Soap has been made in the same way for centuries. The basic ingredients are fat and caustic soda (also know as lye), to which are added extra oils, glycerine, herbs, perfume and colour. Caustic soda is highly alkaline which can upset the skin's natural acid (pH) balance, but skin restores itself to normal within 20 minutes. You can help the process along by adding a few drops of lemon juice or cider vinegar to your final rinse.

The fats in soap combine with the minerals in hard water to form a scum,

Cleansing creams and lotions are all made from oils, waxes and water used in different proportions. To this base can be added various herbs and emollients to make the product more astringent or more moisturizing according to the skin's needs.

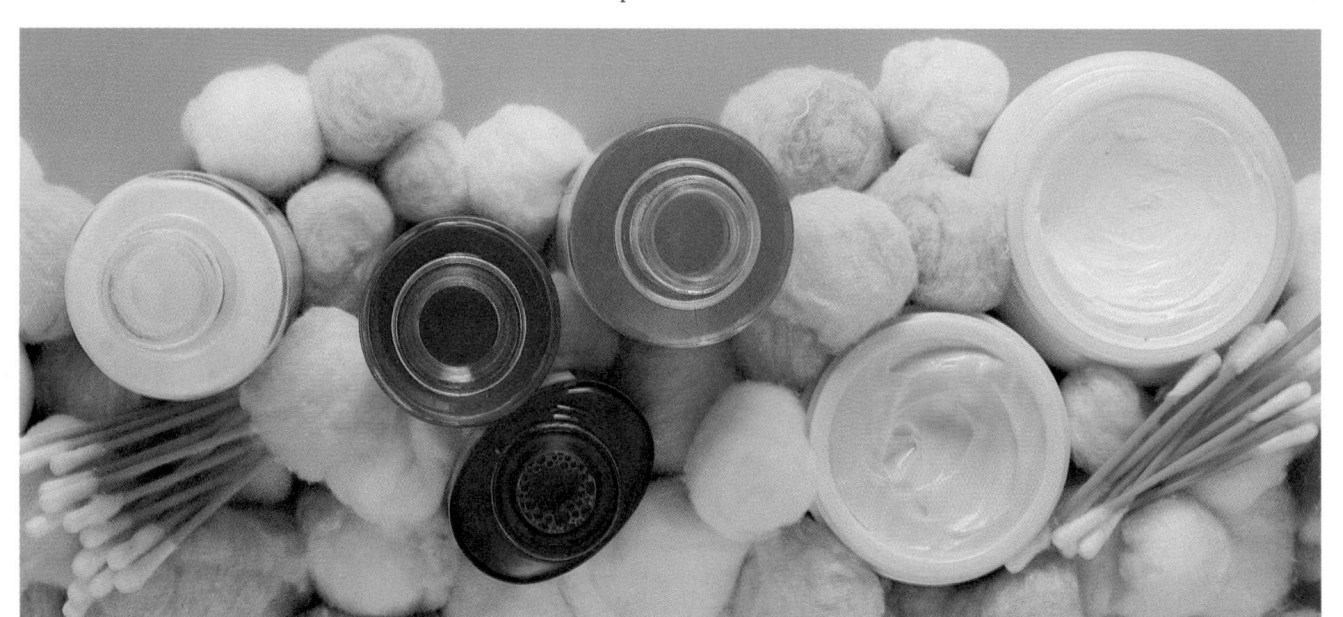

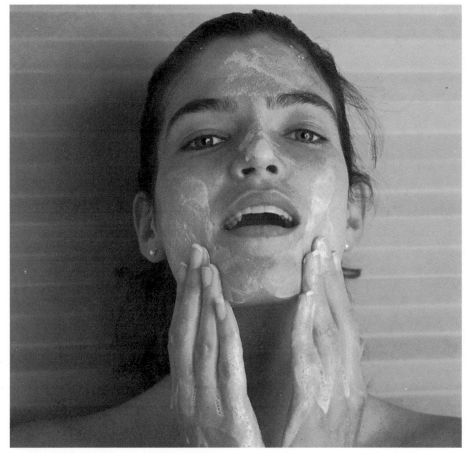

Soaps do a very efficient job of removing
excess oils and grime from the skin, but
creams are better for removing make-up.
Only use the mildest, unperfumed soaps,
and rinse the skin well afterwards with
lukewarm water.

which can be counteracted by adding a pinch of borax to your final rinse.

Liquid soaps and shampoos are detergent instead of soap based. Detergent is a petroleum derivitive which whisks up into a stronger lather and does not make scum. Some detergent products have enough oil and water added to make them gentle on the skin, but others are much harsher than soap. When using any detergent product choose the mildest you can find. When buying commercial soaps the best ones for your skin are 'Castile' or simple soaps, which have no additives and are white and unperfumed. Soaps with added glycerine are also very mild. In the recipe section you will find formulas for making soap from scratch, and also for making soaps by adding herbal ingredients to grated 'Castile' soaps. The purest soap of all is made from the herb soapwort, which is one of nature's own cleansers.

Cleansing creams, milks and lotions

All creams, whether they be for cleansing or moisturizing are made from the same basic mix of oils, waxes and water. The original cold creams contain olive oil, beeswax and rosewater, and they are as pure and pleasant to use as anything you can buy today. These creams are called cold because the evaporation of their water content on contact with the skin gives a cooling

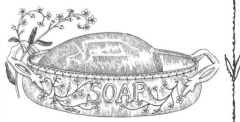

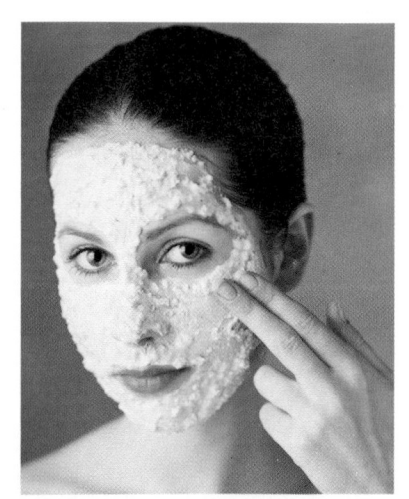

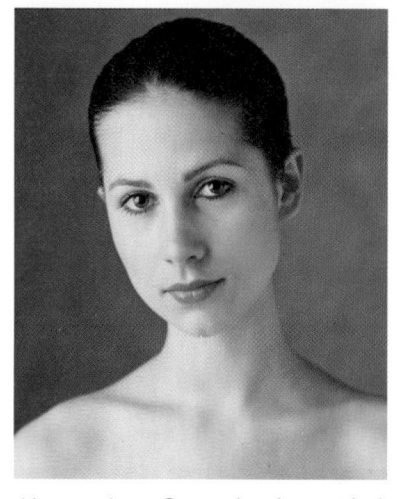

Above and top: Oatmeal makes an ideal gentle skin scrub for ridding the skin of dead skin cells. It is easily made by mixing a couple of tablespoons of oatmeal with water to form a paste, and massaging it gently over the skin. Wash off with warm water.

sensation. Cold cream can be used to cleanse and moisturize. Today's more sophisticated cleansers contain more water to give a more liquid product, so that less of an oily residue is left on the skin. Moisturizers contain refined oils in greater quantity to 'feed' the skin.

Commercial medicated lotion cleansers contain strong antiseptics and alcohol – which can be very hard on the skin. It is far better to use a mild herbal cleanser for problem skins, followed by a natural antiseptic such as witch-hazel dabbed directly on blemishes.

Toners, fresheners and astringents

Skin toners are very useful after using soap or creams because they remove the last residue of these products, leaving the face feeling cool and fresh. Toners, fresheners and astringents contain the same basic ingredients – water, glycerine and alcohol – but in different proportions. Some toners and fresheners are alcohol free, and the best ones contain natural herbal astringents such as witch-hazel, elderflower or camomile. They can also contain lemon or cider vinegar to restore the acid balance to the skin. Alcohol in astringents makes the skin tingle and tighten, as it causes a slight swelling around the pores, making them look smaller. Alcohol is also very efficient at stripping away oil, so it is only recommended as an additive for very greasy skins.

Exfoliators and skin scrubs

Once a week all skins benefit from a gently abrasive scrub to remove dead skin cells that have been lying too long on the skin's surface. This then leaves the skin finer and fresher. The simplest skin scrubs are abrasive substances such as sea salt, oatmeal, ground almonds, orange peel and mashed strawberries. Oily skins benefit from regular exfoliating (another word for cell removal), while dry and sensitive skins will only need treatment once a week.

Deep cleansing with masks and steam treatments

The other once a week activity to maintain perfect skin is an extra deep cleanse with steam, followed by a face mask. The heat and moisture provided by steam softens and relaxes the skin, helping to release ingrained dirt and boosting the blood circulation. Adding herbs to the hot water also helps to aid this cleansing and stimulating action.

A herbal face mask tightens the skin, leaving it looking smooth and refined. Some clay-based masks also act as exfoliators, removing those dingy surface cells. Masks should always be splashed off with cool water to leave the skin looking smooth.

Drawing masks are very beneficial to oily skins, while dry skins enjoy extra-moisturizing masks such as those containing eggs, oils and honey. Avocados make a very nourishing face mask, and bananas and many other fruits are also good. Suit your mask to your needs – when your skin looks blemished and oily choose a deep-cleansing mask, when it seems dry and tired treat it to a moisturizing one.

Dry skins can be revived with a nourishing face mask such as one made from ground almonds, melon, honey and herbs. Pound all the ingredients together and spread evenly over the face, then relax and wait for the mask to do its cleansing work. Wash off thoroughly with warm water.

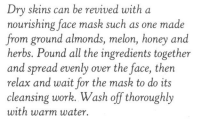

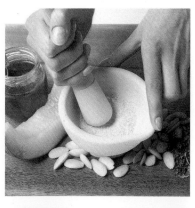

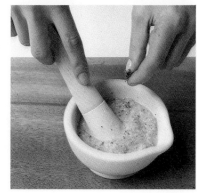

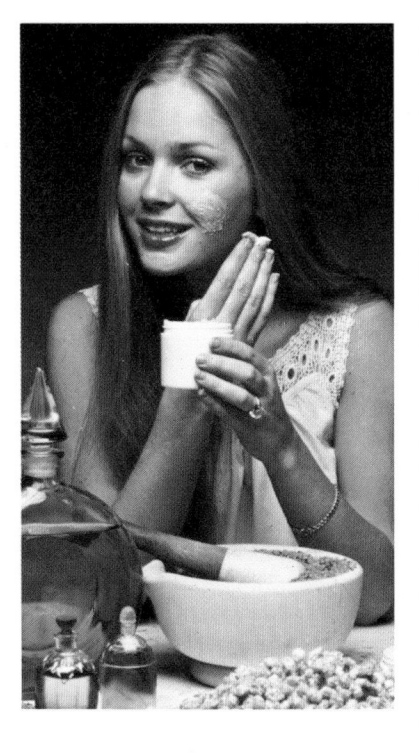

Moisturizers work by placing an oily film over the surface of the skin, so helping the cells to retain moisture. Watch your skin closely and apply moisturizer whenever you feel it is necessary - not only last thing at night and first thing in the morning.

Moisturizing

It is the water content in the skin that keeps it supple and young looking, not the oil content. But oil on the surface of the skin helps the cells to retain this vital moisture, without it evaporating off into the air. The skin's natural oil, sebum, is designed to cope with this task, but it can be unstable in its efficiency. Sometimes the skin produces too much oil, leading to clogged pores, spots and pimples. At other times the skin has too little oil, either because the sebaceous glands are not making enough, or because oil has been stripped from the skin by over-cleansing or harsh weather conditions. This is when a moisturizer is invaluable, because it can duplicate the action of sebum and provide that protective film to stop moisture escaping.

Basic creams made from oil, wax and water cope with this task admirably. Moisturizers also often contain ingredients intended to feed vitamins and proteins into the skin. While dermatologists would argue that it is impossible to get such substances into the skin as this organ is designed to repel all intruders, adding vitamins and proteins in natural substances certainly does not do the skin any harm, and helps it to maintain a smooth, silky appearance. The very latest commercial creams contain collagen and elastin, the proteins responsible for keeping the lower layer of skin (the dermis) supple. These creams are extremely expensive and have no scientific backing to prove their worth. Far better to make your own cheap, but extremely pleasant moisturizers which will fulfil all the same functions as these over-priced creams.

Problem skins

Excess sebum causes the pores on the skin to widen, and spots develop when the ducts carrying the sebum from the glands to the surface of the skin become blocked. This stale sebum traps dead skin cells, and on contact with the air this blocking material becomes blackened, causing blackheads. If these become infected under the surface, pus collects, and a red spot with a head is the result.

It is not possible to slow this flow of excess sebum, so the only solution is to try and keep the pores unblocked, so preventing this build-up.

The simplest way to keep pores clear is to exfoliate the skin regularly, and to dab the pores with a mild antiseptic to stop infection. If blackheads and spots look ready to pop out, you can empty the pore by squeezing the material out. But always steam your face first to relax and soften the skin, and always cover your fingers with tissues to prevent breaking the skin with the pressure from your fingernails, and spreading infection. Afterwards dab the emptied pores with a mild herbal antiseptic.

Other skin problems such as thread veins and uneven pigmentation are harder to treat. But certain hebal remedies are believed to help with these skin irregularities, by helping the blood circulation and mildly bleaching the skin. You will find formulas in the recipe section which are pleasant to try.

The body

The skin in your body from the neck to your feet needs almost as much care as the skin on your face, and the ideal time for top-to-toe skin care is at bath time. The body enjoys being cleansed, toned, exfoliated and moisturized just like the face, and self-massage both relaxes and firms up the figure.

Bathing

Once a day or every other day is an adequate amount of bathing. If you bathe more often you could dehydrate your skin. If you bathe less often stale oil and bacteria will build up on the skin surface, causing perspiration odour. As well as giving your body a thorough cleanse, lying in a warm fragrant bath relaxes your whole system completely. Make your bath really luxurious with additives to soothe, stimulate or soften the skin. In the past wealthy women have used large quantities of exotic substances to bathe in, but simpler and much cheaper to use, are dried herbs and flowers which have soothing or invigorating aromas. Oils added to the bath float on the surface

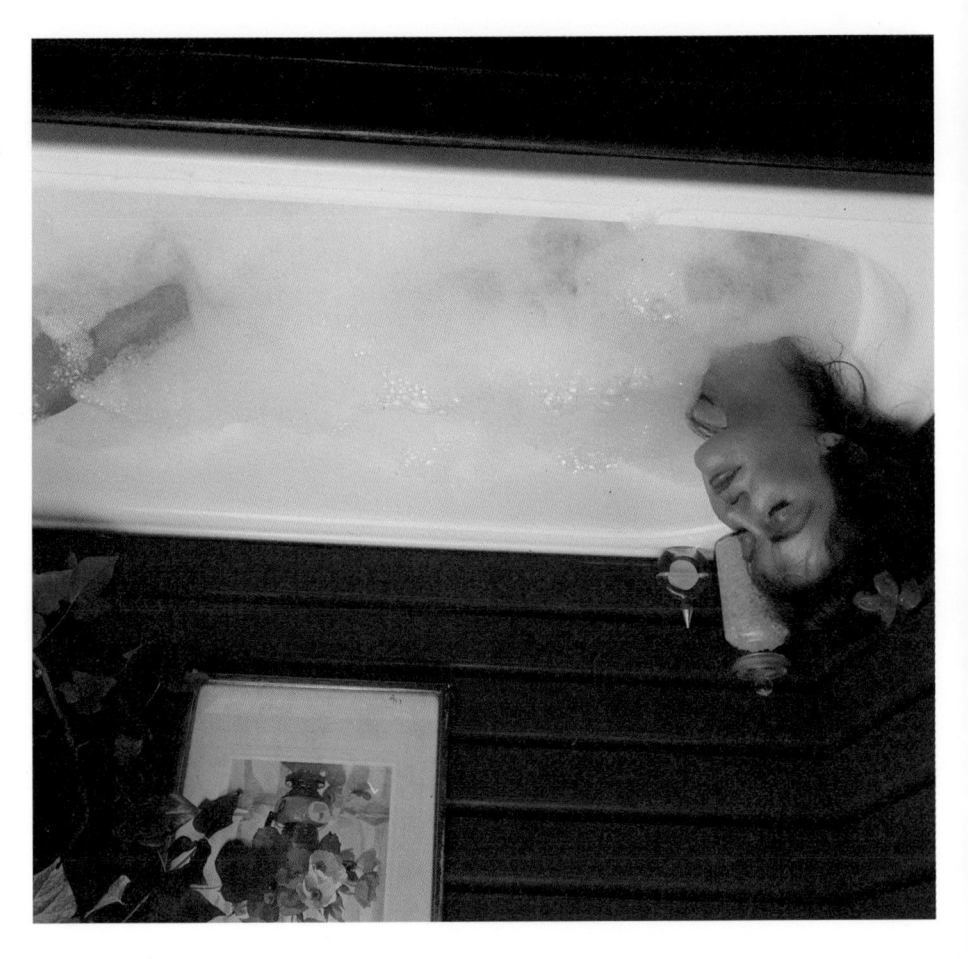

Nothing soothes the body like a long, hot fragrant bath. Fill muslin bags with a selection of herbs and tie them over the hot taps so that the water runs through, or make your own perfumed herbal bubble baths and oils.

and coat your skin as you step out of the bath. Essential oils of flowers can be added to the water to give heavenly, exotic scents. If you prefer the feel of bubble baths, add herbal infusions to a detergent-based, mild commercial product.

Exfoliating the body

Dead skin cells build up on parts of the body like heels, soles of feet, knees and elbows. Rub them away with a loofah or use a grainy scrub containing oatmeal or salt to gently remove them. The backs of thighs, arms and the back also retain some dead cells, although it is not so noticeable, and will benefit from gentle abrasion.

After bath oils

While the skin is still warm and slightly damp, be lavish with the body oil. The action of massaging also helps to firm up the skin, so give your body a thorough going over, concentrating on potentially flabby areas like the thighs and hips. Breasts benefit from gentle massage working upwards from nipples to neck with light, rapid movements. Extracts of plants and flowers can help disperse any unattractive cellulite (the dimpled fat that gathers on thighs and backs of arms) and help sagging breasts regain some firmness and shape.

Body powders

While the skin is warm and relaxed, some dampness may remain between the toes, and under arms and breasts. A soft fragrant powder made from talcum powder and herbs will absorb any remaining moisture.

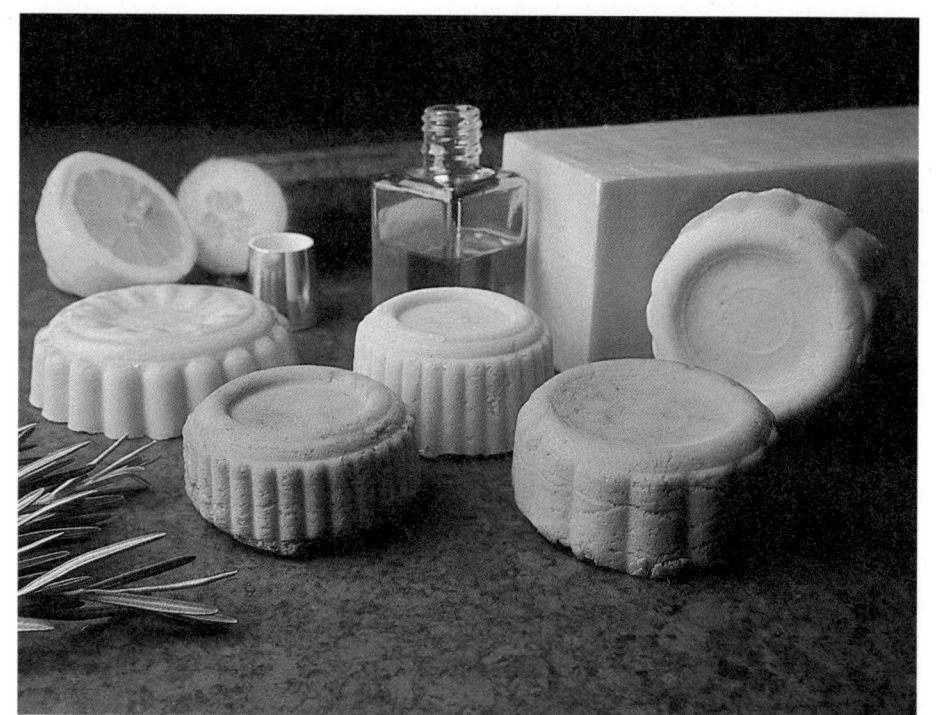

Soap-making is great fun and the finished products make perfect gifts for friends and family. You can make soaps from scratch with lard and caustic soda, or grate down ready-made soap and add the oils and herbs of your choice.

Soaps

Making soap involves the use of caustic soda, which can be a little daunting as the fumes are heavy and the mixture can burn you if it touches your skin. But if you are careful when handling this ingredient and wear plastic gloves there is little reason to fear accident. Soap is made by the chemical reaction between caustic soda, water and lard. Once you have your basic mixture you can add extra oils, fruits and perfume to it. Quantities must be followed exactly and temperatures controlled. The fat and caustic soda solution are heated separately then mixed together. They interact and form a thick cream. This is poured into moulds and left to harden for several weeks.

Equipment Caustic soda damages metals, so use only stainless steel or enamel pots for heating the mixtures, and glass for mixing the caustic soda with water. Soap moulds can be plastic or wood, lined with greaseproof paper or damp muslin to stop soap sticking.

Skin and the sun

The cult of the suntan is a fairly recent phenomenon – only 50 years ago a woman could not be too pale, and a dark tan was thought highly vulgar. With today's fascination with foreign travel, a tan is considered a status symbol and generally thought very attractive indeed.

A touch of sun does everyone good, giving the skin and hair a glow they lack in cold winter months. But a suntan is actually the sign of skin protecting itself against damage, and is not a sign of healthy skin at all. Too much sun does irreparable harm to skin, drying it out and breaking down the collagen fibres, leaving skin wrinkled and loose. Seek a compromise with your sunbathing and achieve that attractive golden glow without having to pay for it later.

It is the sun's ultra-violet rays that penetrate the skin, and force it to produce increased amounts of the brown pigment melanin to protect itself against sunburn. How much melanin you produce is determined by how many melanin cells you were born with, and this melanin quota can not be artificially stimulated. If you are naturally dark-skinned you will tan deeply and easily, but if you are pale-skinned too much exposure to the sun is bound to make you burn. Only the foolhardy insist on sunbathing when they are naturally pale. Far better to accept your skin's chemistry and aim for a light, golden glow. It is only fashion, not aesthetics that decrees that brown is more beautiful!

Tanning lotions and after-sun treatments

All skin types should keep their skins well-oiled in the sun to prevent excessive moisture loss. Several plant extracts are renowned for their tan enhancing and protecting qualities, notably coconut oil, bergamot oil and aloe vera. You will find recipes for all of these in the following sections.

Sunshine in highly concentrated doses can leave even the darkest skins sore and tingling. Cooling after-sun preparations containing cucumber, calamine, comfrey and yoghurt are all excellent to relieve the discomfort.

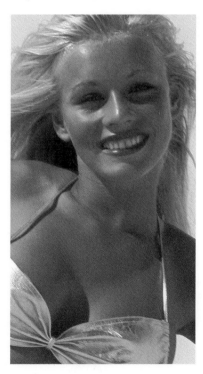

Many people consider a suntan a highly desirable beauty asset. The sun can add a glow of health to both skin and hair, but sunbathing should only be enjoyed in moderation as too much sun can do irreparable damage to the skin.

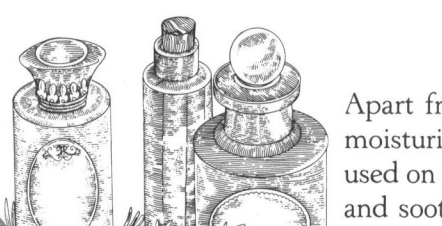

Perfumes and pot pourri

Apart from their healing properties and abilities to cleanse, stimulate and moisturize, plants are delightful to use for their fragrance alone. Perfumes used on the neck, body and wrist make you smell wonderful and they can lift and soothe the spirits, too. Famous perfumes are masterpieces of skill and imagination, as well as complicated blending techniques. But you can make your own pleasant-smelling colognes and pot pourri using the same basic ingredients.

Perfumes

Commercial perfumes come in the form of concentrated perfume, parfum de toilette, eau-de-cologne and solid perfume.

Perfume in its most concentrated form is made up of 15-25 per cent flower and plant oils, and 75-85 per cent alcohol. Parfum de toilette is the next strongest with 12-15 per cent perfume, some alcohol and distilled water. Eau-de-cologne is the weakest with only 2-6 per cent perfume, water and alcohol. Solid perfumes contain perfume suspended in a wax and oil base.

Commercial perfumes also contain fixatives to reduce the rate of evaporation of the fragrance. These are often animal derivitives such as ambergris, musk and civet. Synthetic fixatives are becoming increasingly popular. You can use a herbal alternative in the form of benzoin, orris root, clove or lavender oil.

Making eau-de-colognes and flower waters

The simplest way to make an eau-de-cologne or flower water is first to make an essence. You do this by dissolving a small amount of the essential oil of a herb or flower in a larger amount of alcohol. Use 15ml (½fl oz or 1 tablespoon) of essential oil to 450ml (¾pt) of alcohol. You then add water to dilute the perfumed alcohol (or cologne) to make a flower water. Half a teaspoon of the cologne added to 300ml (½ pt) of purified water makes a cheap flower water to use as lavishly as you want.

Pot pourri

Dried flowers, leaves and seeds can be used in their entire state to create heady, fragrant mixtures ideal for scenting drawers, cupboards or even entire rooms. The most fragrant and colourful flowers and leaves are chosen, then carefully dried away from the light to retain maximum colour and scent. When dry, essential oils and fixatives are added to stop the fragrance evaporating away. Pot pourri mixtures can be ground down into fine powders and sewn into sachets of muslin to scent drawers. Pot pourri should be contained in glass or china pots, and placed around the room.

Any aromatic plants can be included in pot pourri, so choose from flowers, herbs, fruits, barks and spices. It gives the mixture an identity to

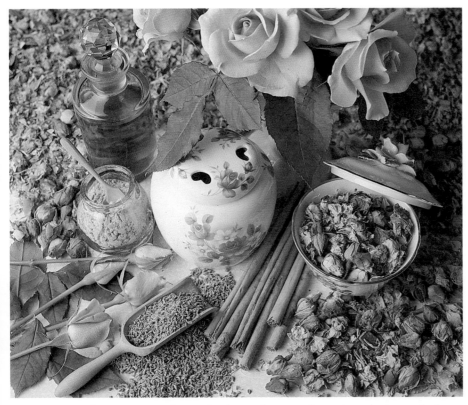

Pot pourri and perfumed sachets are simple to make, and delightful to use. Roses make a popular base for pot pourri mixture as they retain a lot of their distinctive fragrance when dried, and they also mix well with other herbs and spices.

have a main fragrance, and rose or lavender are the most obvious choices. The dried petals should be placed in an air-tight container and covered with a thin layer of salt and orris root mixed. This both helps to dry them further and fix the scent. After a few hours, add another layer of petals, and another layer of salt and orris root. Keep layering until you are satisfied with the mix, then add your dried ingredients and your essential oils. Stir well and cover tightly, then leave to mature for a few weeks.

There are no rules about combinations of colour and fragrance, but here are some to try. Be careful with the quantities of oil, salt and orris. For a simple pot pourri use 3 cups each of dried rose petals, rosemary leaves and lavender flowers, 2 tablespoons orange and lemon peel, 2 crushed cinnamon sticks, 1 tablespoon crushed cloves, 3 tablespoons ground orris root, 2 tablespoons salt and 6 drops of geranium, bergamot and sandalwood oil.

For fragrance

Basil, bay, balm, marjoram, mint, sweet pea, rose, rosemary, jasmine, rose geranium, carnations, honeysuckle, lavender, pinks verbena, gardenias, cinnamon, clove, thyme, coriander seeds, nutmeg, orange and lemon peel.

For colour

Rose, lavender, lilac, violet, marigold, pansy.

Essential oils

Lavender, rose, geranium, bergamot, lemon, orange, patchouli, sandalwood.

Cleansers, toners and moisturizers

The following soaps, cleansers, fresheners and masks featured here can all be made simply with readily available ingredients and do not need a full recipe. Detailed recipes follow on page. 76.

Soap

The basic soap recipe is on page 76. Any of these ingredients can be added for perfume, colour or moisturizing effects.

Perfume oils Add a few drops of any oil of your choice. Geranium, camomile, jasmine, lavender, verbena, orange blossom and sandalwood all smell delicious.

Colour Use just a couple of drops of food colourings to make your soap look more attractive. Pink and green look effective. For yellow use an infusion of saffron, made by putting a teaspoon of saffron in a cup of boiling purified water. Leave to stand for 2 days, and then use a few drops.

Fruits and grains can add texture and moisture. Add 2 tablespoons of mashed avocado, cucumber, strawberry, honey, ground almonds, soaked oatmeal or bran.

Glycerine Add two tablespoons of glycerine at the start of the thickening process for an extra silky, gentle soap.

Making soap with castile soap flakes You can bypass the caustic soda stage of soap making by using ready-made simple, unperfumed soap. Use plain soap flakes or grate down bars of white soap, then add the herb of your choice – yarrow, parsley, fennel, honeysuckle and rosemary are all particularly good herbs to use.

Simple cleansers

Oils, milk, herbal infusions and fruit and vegetable juices can all be used as simple cleansers. Make-up needs to be dissolved by an oil and wax cream, but basic natural ingredients cope well with everyday grime.

Oils. Almond, avocado and sunflower oil are all light oils to use. Smooth on with the fingers and tissue off.

Milks. Whole milk, buttermilk and yoghurt all make good cleansers used straight on cotton wool. Or mix them with herbal and vegetable waters for a lighter consistency.

Herbal infusions (see p.20). Elderflower, balm, yarrow, cowslip and verbena all make good cleansing infusions. Use them alone or added to milks.

Fruits and vegetables. Strawberry juice, cucumber juice, lemon juice and potato water all make efficient cleansers used alone or in conjunction with other ingredients.

Simple skin fresheners

These should be made up for each application.

Lemon juice squeezed in water.

Cider vinegar. Add a teaspoon to a cup of water to restore acid mantle to skin after washing with soap.

Camphor. Two drops in a cup of water.

Cucumber, liquidize 1 cucumber and strain juice into a saucepan. Heat to simmering, skim away froth. Bottle and keep chilled in fridge.

Herbal infusions

These make ideal skin fresheners used on their own. Make a mild infusion (25g [1oz] of one of the ingredients listed to 600ml (1 pint) of purified water and let steep for at least 2 hours before straining and bottling in large bottle. Keep chilled in fridge. Adding a few drops of tincture of benzoin or myrrh will make the herbal freshener slightly more astringent for oily skins, and help to preserve the infusion.

Greasy skins
Yarrow infusion
Parsley infusion
Mint infusion
Fennel infusion
Sage infusion
Blackberry leaves infusion

Dry skins
Rosemary infusion
Comfrey infusion
Camomile infusion
Honeysuckle infusion
Angelica infusion
Rose infusion

Sallow and freckled skins
Tansy infusion
Dandelion infusion

Masks

The following natural ingredients make ideal face masks when used just on their own.

Yoghurt mask (for removing blackheads)
Smooth plain yoghurt over the face and leave for 15 minutes. Rinse off with cool water.

Fruit and vegetable masks
Many fruits and vegetables make ideal skin masks used alone or in conjunction with other ingredients.

Strawberries, mash 3 and spread over the skin.

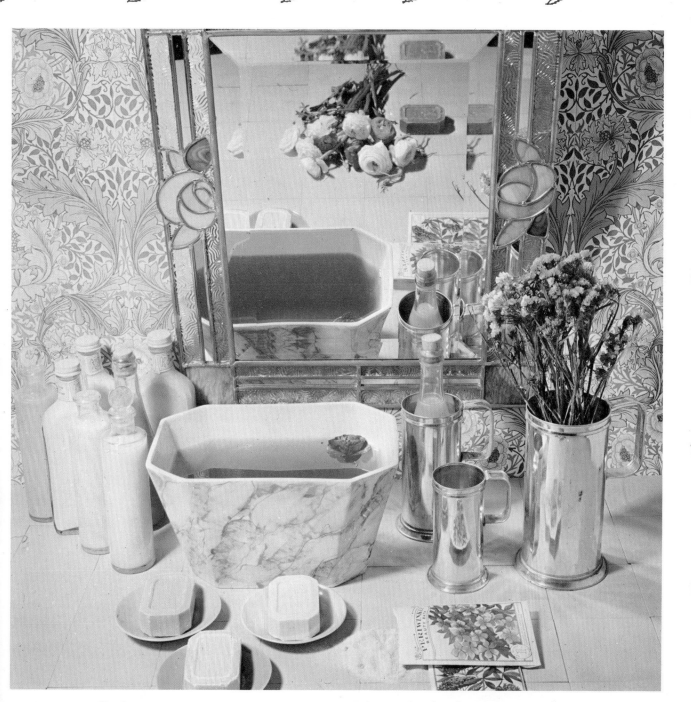

Peach, mash a half and use.

Tomato, mash one and combine with oatmeal to make a paste.

Apple, grate and apply on gauze as a poultice (gauze side against the skin).

Potato, extract the juice (using an extractor) and mix with enough kaolin to make a paste.

Melon, mash and apply on gauze as a poultice.

Papaya, mash ½ of a firm fruit and use 2 tablespoons as a mask.

Avocado, mash ½ a ripe fruit and mix with a teaspoon of honey and a squeeze of lemon.

Banana, mash and mix with a teaspoon of honey and a little ground almond to make a paste.

Basic soap
(Makes 4 bars)
4 cups of lard
2 cups of purified water
5 tablespoons of caustic soda crystals

Prepare the caustic soda solution by pouring the water into a large glass bowl and adding the caustic soda, stirring it with a wooden spoon until it dissolves. It does not need to be heated as a great deal of heat is generated by the soda alone. Test it with a thermometer – it will be ready to use when it has cooled to around 32°C (90°F). While the caustic soda is cooling, melt the lard in a saucepan. Remove from the heat and cool to the same temperature as the caustic soda. With the lard off the heat, add the caustic soda very, very slowly. Stir with a wooden spoon. The first sign that a reaction is taking place is that the lard turns pink as its chemical mixture is broken down, then it will gradually turn white. Stir slowly all the time, for about 30 minutes, taking occasional breaks. When the mixture resembles a thick custard, pour into the moulds. Perfume, colour and oils need to be added after the soap has thickened, but before pouring it into the moulds. Stir them in well to ensure they are evenly mixed. Cover the moulds with a towel to stop them drying too fast, and keep in a warm dry place such as the airing cupboard. They will take at least two weeks to set, longer with added ingredients.

Herbal castile soap
(Makes 4 bars)
450g (1lb) soap flakes
2 cups strong (use 50g [2oz] of herbs) herbal infusion (see p. 20)
Few drops perfume oil
Colouring

Melt the soap flakes and chosen herbal infusion in an enamel saucepan over a gentle heat, stirring continuously. Take off the heat and when the mixture has cooled a little, add the perfume oil and colouring. Pour into moulds and leave to dry for a few weeks.
Herbal additives Some herbs contain more mucilage than others, and will produce a softer soap, e.g. comfrey, houseleek and marshmallow.
Honey and lanolin can be added to the soap flakes to make a soft soap. Reduce the amount of soap flakes accordingly.

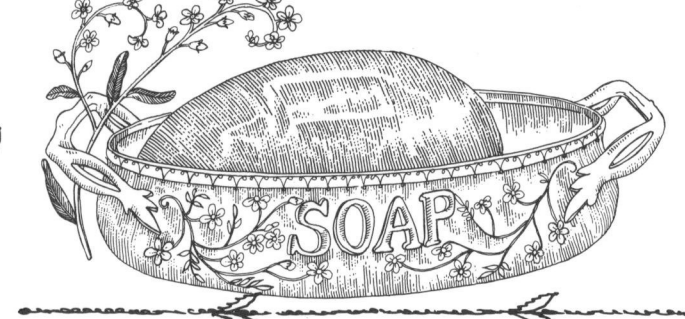

Honey and comfrey soap
(Makes 4 bars)
250g (9oz) soap flakes
2 cups strong (50g [2oz] of herb) comfrey infusion (see p. 20)
125g (4oz) honey
Few drops verbena oil

Melt the soap flakes and comfrey infusion in one saucepan over a gentle heat, the honey in another. Add the honey to the soap mixture, stirring continuously. Take off the stove and as the mixture cools, add the verbena oil. Pour into moulds and leave to dry for several weeks as before.

Oatmeal and lavender soap
(Makes 4 bars)
250g (9oz) soap flakes
2 cups lavender infusion (see p.20)
50g (2oz) oatmeal
Few drops lavender oil

Add the soap flakes to the lavender infusion and heat together and once the soap flakes have melted, add the oatmeal, stirring well. Take off the heat and as the mixture cools add the lavender oil. Pour into moulds. This gritty soap is a good exfoliator. Make it with rosewater and geranium oil, instead of the lavender infusion and oil, for variety.

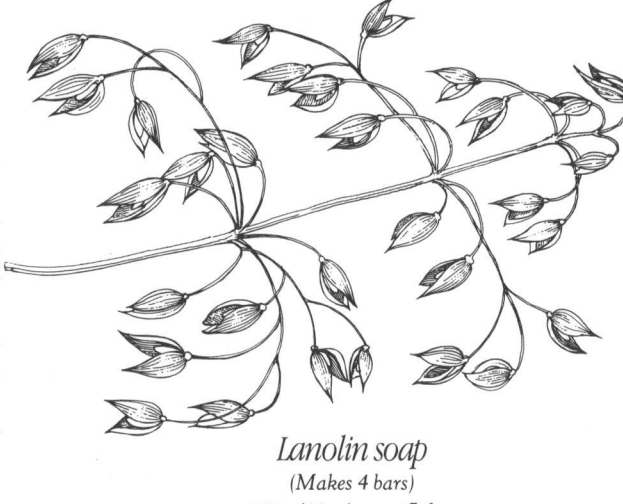

Lanolin soap
(Makes 4 bars)
350g (12oz) soap flakes
125g (4oz) lanolin
2 cups rosewater
Few drops geranium oil
Few drops of pink colouring

Melt the lanolin in a double boiler or in a heat-resistant bowl over hot water. Heat the soap flakes and rosewater separately, then add the soap mixture to the lanolin in a thin stream, beating hard. As the mixture cools, add the perfume oil, and colouring. Pour into moulds.

Elderflower cleansing milk
(1 medium bottle)
3 tablespoons elderflowers
300ml (½ pt) buttermilk

Heat the flowers in the milk until nearly boiling, then turn down and simmer for half an hour. Leave covered for 2 hours, then strain. Keep chilled in the fridge. Apply using cotton wool. This cleanser is particularly good for dry skin.

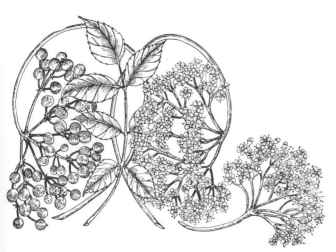

Cucumber cleansing milk
(1 medium bottle)
¼ ripe cucumber
150ml (¼ pt) milk

Slice and blend the cucumber and press through a sieve, or use a juice extractor. Add to the milk, bottle, and keep chilled in fridge. When using, apply to cotton wool and wipe over the face. Only make this cleanser in small amounts as it will only keep a few days. Ideal for an oily skin.

Almond milk
(1 medium bottle)
4 tablespoons ground almonds
300 ml (½ pt) buttermilk

Add the almonds to the milk, heat and simmer for half an hour. Leave covered for two hours then strain and bottle. Keep chilled, and apply using cotton wool. A good cleanser for dry skin.

Yoghurt and lemon cleansing milk
(1 application)
1 tablespoon natural yoghurt
1 teaspoon lemon juice

Simply mix the two ingredients together. Ideal for oily skin.

Basic light cleansing cream
(1 small pot)
15g (½oz) emulsifying wax
6 tablespoons almond oil
¼ teaspoon borax
5 tablespoons rosewater

Melt the wax in a double boiler or in a heat-resistant bowl over hot water. When melted add the almond oil and stir together. Warm the rosewater separately, and dissolve the borax in it. Remove the oil and wax mixture from the heat and add the rosewater mixture in a trickle, whisking hard until it thickens to a soft white cream. Scoop into a labelled pot.

When using, massage into the face with your fingertips and wipe off with tissues. To make variations on this basic cream add a herbal infusion (see p.20) such as yarrow or verbena. You can also add a few drops of perfume oil at the cooling stage.

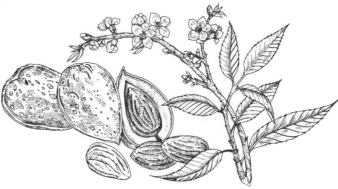

Cocoa butter and lanolin cleanser
(1 small pot)
½ tablespoon cocoa butter
½ tablespoon lanolin
4 tablespoons almond oil
2 tablespoons rosewater
¼ teaspoon borax

Melt the butter, lanolin and oil together in a double boiler or in a heat-resistant bowl over hot water. Heat the rosewater separately with the borax, remove ingredients from heat and whisk together. Pour into a pot and label. This oily cleanser is very gentle on dry or ageing skin.

Avocado cleansing cream

(1 small pot)

15g (½oz) emulsifying wax
1 teaspoon lanolin
6 tablespoons avocado oil
4 tablespoons purified water

Melt the wax and lanolin in a double boiler or a heat-resistant bowl over hot water, then stir in the oil. Gently warm the purified water. Remove the wax and oil mixture from the heat and add the warm water, whisking into a cream. Pour into a pot and label. Ideal for dry skin.

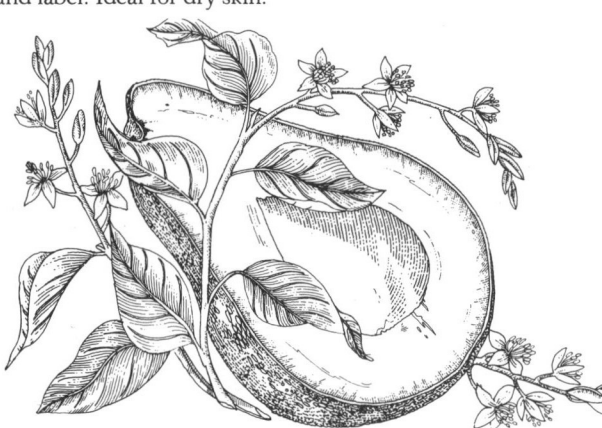

Cucumber and yarrow cleanser

(1 small pot)

1 teaspoon emulsifying wax
4 tablespoons almond oil
¼ cucumber, liquidized and strained
6 tablespoons (use 15g [½oz] of herb) yarrow infusion (see p.20)
3 drops tincture of benzoin

Melt the wax in a double boiler or a heat-resistant bowl over hot water and add the almond oil. Heat 2 tablespoons of the cucumber juice with the yarrow infusion and add to the oil and whisk mixture away from the heat. Beat hard. Add the benzoin stir in, and put in a pot and label. Keep chilled in the fridge. This cleanser is good for oily skin.

Rosewater and witch hazel toner

(1 medium bottle)

150ml (¼ pint) rosewater
150ml (¼ pint) witch hazel

Simply pour both ingredients into a bottle and shake together. Altering the proportions can match your skin type. More witch hazel will make a more astringent mix for oily skins, more

rosewater a milder one for dry skins. For very dry skins add a few drops of glycerine to the toner mixture as this makes a very soothing addition.

Elderflower freshener

(1 small bottle)

3 tablespoons elderflower infusion (see p.20)
3 tablespoons rosewater
3 tablespoons witch hazel
1 teaspoon borax

Shake all the ingredients together thoroughly in a small bottle. Elderflowers are particularly renowned for their skin softening and whitening properties.

Marigold astringent

(1 medium bottle)

6 tablespoons marigold infusion (see p.20)
2 tablespoons witch hazel
Few drops tincture of benzoin
or ½ teaspoon alum

Shake all the ingredients together in a bottle. This astringent is also particularly helpful for problem skins.

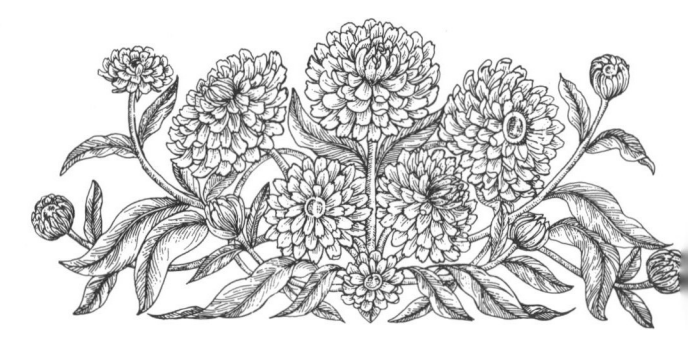

Sage astringent

(1 medium bottle)

4 tablespoons dried sage
6 tablespoons vodka
¼ teaspoon borax
3 tablespoons witch hazel
1 teaspoon glycerine

Macerate the sage in the vodka for 2 weeks then strain. Dissolve the borax in the witch hazel and add this to the vodka, stir in the glycerine. Pour into a bottle, shake and use. This is ideal for helping to combat oily skin.

Oatmeal scrub (for delicate skin)
(1 application)
1 tablespoon fine oatmeal
Milk to make a paste

Mix the ingredients together and massage over the face, paying particular attention to oily areas. Rinse off with warm water.

Sugar scrub
(For oily skin)
(1 application)
soap
1 tablespoon sugar

As you lather up your usual soap, add the tablespoon of sugar. Massage into the face and rinse well with warm water. Finish with a lemon juice or cider vinegar freshener (see p.74).

Almond scrub
(For dry skin)
(1 application)

1 tablespoon ground almonds
Melted honey or sunflower oil to make a paste

Mix the two ingredients together and massage gently all over the face. Wash off with a flannel warmed in water.

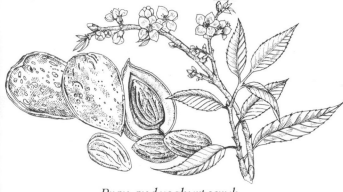

Bran and yoghurt scrub
(For blemished skin)
(1 application)
2 tablespoons bran
1 tablespoon sea salt
Yoghurt to make a paste

Mix dry ingredients together then add the yoghurt to make a paste. This is a good scrub for blemished skins, but use gentle massage movements to apply it.

Oatmeal and orange scrub
(For normal skin)
(1 application)
1 tablespoon finely ground oatmeal
1 tablespoon dried and ground orange peel
1 tablespoon ground almonds
Milk to make a paste

Mix the dry ingredients together and add the milk to make a paste. Massage into the skin, rinse off with warm water.

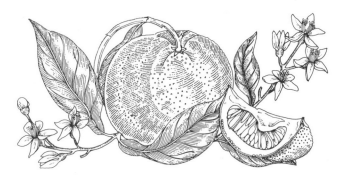

Wheatgerm and cream scrub
(For dry skin)
(1 application)
1 tablespoon wheatgerm
1 tablespoon cream

Mix the ingredients together to make a smooth paste and massage into the skin. This is a very gentle scrub for dry or particularly sensitive skins.

Steam treatments
(1 application)
A large bowl of steaming water
1 tablespoon camomile
1 tablespoon lavender
1 tablespoon elderflower
1 tablespoon comfrey
1 tablespoon rosemary
1 tablespoon thyme

Add the herbs to the water then lean your face over the bowl with a towel over your head to trap the steam. Keep your face 46cm (18in) away from the steam for a few minutes. Afterwards examine face in a strong light and carefully remove any blackheads with a tissue. A steam treatment is very stimulating and cleansing for the face and helps to soften the skin. After the treatment apply a face mask.

Clay masks
(for oily skins)
(1 application)
**2 teaspoons strong (use 300ml [½pt] to 25g [1oz] herb) herbal
infusion of comfrey, camomile, sage or parsley (see p.20)
2 tablespoons kaolin powder**

Add the kaolin to the herbal infusion of your choice and stir
into a thick paste. Spread the mask over the face and neck and
leave to dry for five to ten minutes. Splash off with tepid water
and pat skin dry with a towel This is a good drawing mask which
removes impurities from the skin.

Yoghurt and yeast mask
(To clear the skin)
(1 application)
**1 tablespoon yoghurt
1 tablespoon powdered brewers' yeast
1 teaspoon lemon juice
1 teaspoon olive oil**

Mix all the ingredients together and smooth over the skin. Leave
on for 15 minutes and then rinse off with cool water. If your skin
is oily, omit the olive oil.

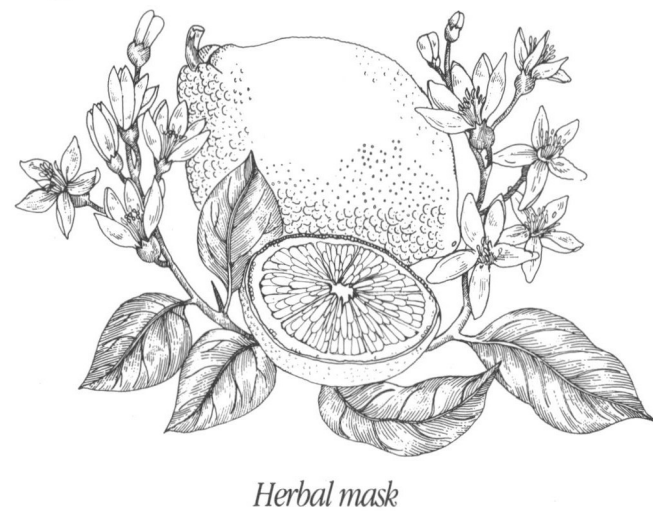

Herbal mask
(For tired skin)
(1 application)
**1 tablespoon fresh comfrey leaves (dried leaves are not suitable)
1 teaspoon of honey
Wheatgerm to make a paste**

Pound the comfrey leaves (or any other fresh herb) into a mush
and stir in the honey and wheatgerm to make a paste. Smooth on
the face and leave on for 10 minutes, splash off with cool water.

Honey and lecithin nourishing mask
(1 application)
**2 tablespoons honey
2 tablespoons cream
2 egg yolks
½ teaspoon cider vinegar
Powdered lecithin to make a paste**

Whisk the wet ingredients together, then add the lecithin to
make a paste. Smooth over the face and leave for 15 minutes,
splash off with cool water.

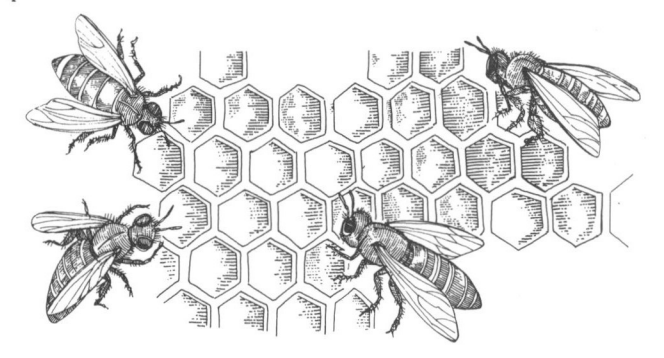

Cucumber mask
(To tighten skin)
(1 application)
**¼ peeled cucumber
½ teaspoon lemon juice
1 teaspoon witch hazel
1 whipped egg white**

Blend the cucumber to a pulp and add the lemon juice and witch
hazel. Pour into a bowl and add the whipped egg white. Smooth
on to the face and allow to dry for 15 minutes. Wipe off with a
warm flannel.

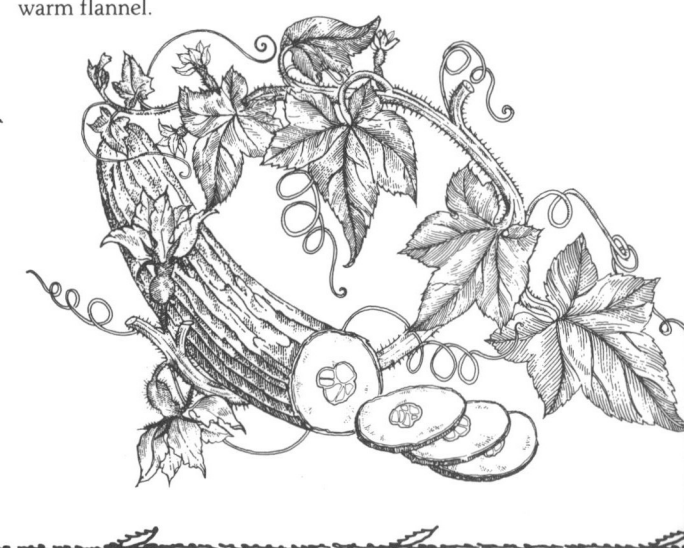

Basic moisturizing cream
(1 pot)

½ tablespoon grated beeswax
1 tablespoon emulsifying wax
4 tablespoons almond oil
2 tablespoons coconut oil
3 tablespoons rosewater
¼ teaspoon borax
Few drops of geranium oil

Melt the waxes together in an enamel double boiler, or in a heat-resistant glass bowl over hot water. Add the oils and stir until smooth. Heat the rosewater separately and add the borax, stirring to dissolve. Take the wax and oil mixture from the heat and stir in the rosewater, a trickle at a time. Beat vigorously or use an electric whisk on slow speed until a smooth white cream forms. As it cools add the essential oil (omit this if your skin is sensitive). Scoop into a pot and label.

This smooth white cream sinks rapidly into the skin leaving it feeling smooth and soft. Instead of the rosewater you could use 3 tablespoons of any herbal infusion (see p.20) of your choice. Add a few drops of tincture of benzoin as a preservative.

Strawberry moisturizer
(1 pot)

2 teaspoons emulsifying wax
2 teaspoons coconut oil
4 teaspoons almond oil
3 tablespoons strawberry juice
Few drops tincture of benzoin
Few drops strawberry essence

Melt the waxes and oils together in a double boiler or a heat-resistant bowl over hot water. Warm the strawberry juice separately then add to the oil mixture away from the heat. As it cools stir in the benzoin and the strawberry perfume essence. Scoop into pot and label. This is a moisturizer for oily skins.

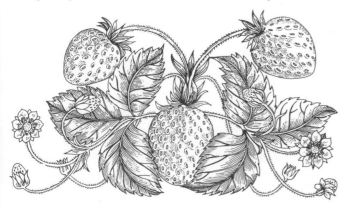

Lanolin and cocoa butter moisturizer
(1 pot)

1 tablespoon emulsifying wax
1 teaspoon lanolin
1 teaspoon cocoa butter
1 tablespoons coconut oil
4 tablespoons rosewater
½ teaspoon borax

Melt the wax, lanolin, cocoa butter and oil together in a double boiler or a heat-resistant bowl over hot water. Warm the rosewater and dissolve the borax in it and then add to the oil mixture away from the heat, a drop at a time. Beat until the cream cools, scoop into a pot and label.

This is an oily moisturizer for dry skins. If you are allergic to lanolin use 2 teaspoons of cocoa butter, if you are allergic to cocoa butter use 2 teaspoons of lanolin. If neither suits your skin, substitute almond oil.

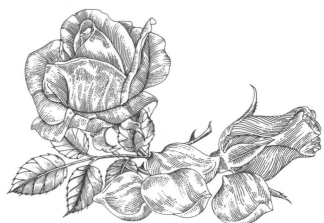

Comfrey moisturizer
(1 pot)

2 teaspoons beeswax
1 teaspoon emulsifying wax
5 teaspoons almond oil
4 tablespoons strong (use 50g [2oz] of herb) comfrey infusion (see p.20)
Few drops tincture of benzoin

Melt the waxes in a double boiler or a heat-resistant bowl over hot water and add the oil. Heat the strained comfrey infusion separately, and beat into the oil mixture away from the heat. Add a few drops of tincture of benzoin as it cools. Stir well and scoop into a pot and label.

This soft, pale brown cream is soothing and healing for dry skins. Add a pleasant fragrance by using a few drops of perfume oil. Marshmallow or lime infusions would make good herb substitutes here.

Marigold moisturizer
(1 pot)
1 teaspoon emulsifying wax
1 teaspoon beeswax
3 tablespoons almond oil
3 tablespoons marigold infusion (see p.20)
Few drops tincture of benzoin

Melt the waxes in a double boiler or a heat-resistant bowl over hot water and add the lanolin. When it has melted, add the oil. Heat the marigold infusion separately, and add in a trickle to the oil and wax away from the heat, beating until creamy. Add the tincture of benzoin as the mixture cools and scoop into pot and label. This is a very pleasant moisturizing cream which is suitable for all skin types.

Avocado cream
(1 pot)
1 teaspoon beeswax
2 teaspoons emulsifying wax
8 teaspoons almond oil
4 teaspoons avocado oil
6 teaspoons rosewater
pinch of borax
perfume oil

Melt the waxes in a double boiler or a heat-resistant bowl over hot water and add the oils. Heat the rosewater separately and dissolve the borax in it. Take the oil and wax mixture off the heat and beat in the rosewater a little at a time. When cool add a perfume oil of your own choice for fragrance and scoop into pot and label.

To make a creamier moisturizer you could also add a teaspoon of peeled and mashed avocado to the heated oils and waxes, before mixing with the rosewater. This is a good moisturizer for oily skins.

Wheatgerm night cream
(1 pot)
1 teaspoon beeswax
1 teaspoon emulsifying wax
1 teaspoon lanolin
4 tablespoons wheatgerm oil
3 tablespoons purified water
¼ teaspoon borax

Melt waxes and lanolin together in a double boiler or a heat-resistant bowl over hot water, then add the oil. Heat the water separately, dissolve the borax in it and add to the oil mixture a drop at a time away from the heat. Scoop into pot and lable. This is a rich night cream for dry skins.

Honey and lecithin skin food
(1 pot)
2 teaspoons lanolin
2 tablespoons sesame oil
½ tablespoon honey
2 tablespoons purified water
1 teaspoon lecithin powder

Melt the lanolin and add the oil and honey. Heat the water separately and add to the oils away from the heat. Let the mixture cool a little and then stir in the lecithin. Scoop into a pot and label. This is an ideal night skin food for tired skins.

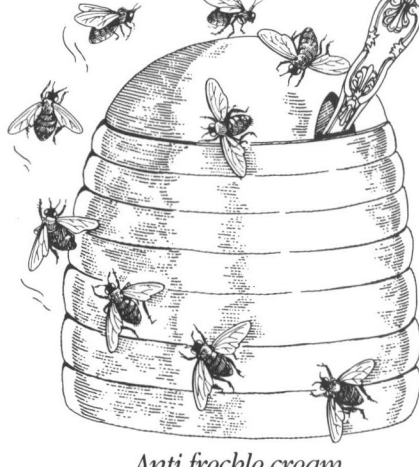

Anti-freckle cream
(1 application)
4 tablespoons buttermilk
1 teaspoon grated horseradish
1 tablespoon fine oatmeal

Mix together the buttermilk and the horseradish and add the oatmeal to make a paste and apply over the freckles. Leave on for 30 minutes and wash off. Repeat once or twice a week.

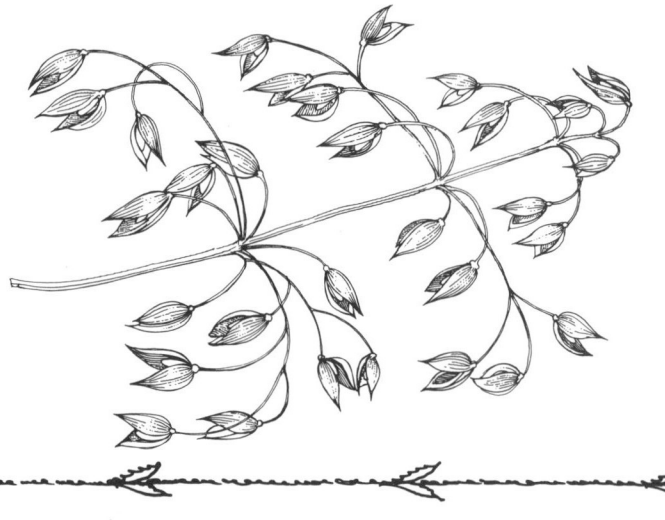

Elderflower anti-freckle lotion
(1 application)
4 tablespoons strong (use 50g [2oz] of herb) elderflower infusion
(p.20)
1 tablespoon lemon juice
½ teaspoon alum

Mix the infusion and the lemon juice together. Apply to freckled areas using cotton wool. Leave for 30 minutes then rinse off. Repeat frequently.

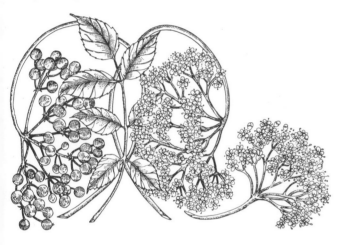

Lettuce thread vein lotion
(1 application)
6 dark green lettuce leaves
½ pint of milk
3 drops tincture of benzoin

Cover the lettuce leaves with the milk and simmer on the stove for half an hour, covered. Allow to cool, still covered, then strain. Add the benzoin and put in a small bottle. Use as a lotion on cotton wool.

Marigold and wheatgerm cream
(for thread veins)
(1 small pot)
2 teaspoons beeswax
1 teaspoon emulsifying wax
5 teaspoons wheatgerm oil
6 tablespoons marigold infusion (see p.20)

Melt the waxes together in a double boiler or a heat-resistant bowl over hot water and add the oil. Heat the marigold infusion separately and add to the oil and wax away from the heat, beating hard, then scoop into a small pot and label. This is a light, creamy lotion for everyday use.

Basic lip salve
(Makes 1 pot)
2 teaspoons beeswax
4 teaspoons almond oil
1 teaspoon rosewater

Melt the beeswax in a double boiler or a heat-resistant bowl over hot water and add the oil and rosewater. Pour into a small pot while it is still warm, where it will set into a white glossy lip salve.

Cocoa butter lip salve
(1 small pot)
2 teaspoons beeswax
1 teaspoon cocoa butter
1 teaspoon almond oil
1 teaspoon rosewater

Melt wax and butter in a double boiler or a heat-resistant bowl over hot water and add the oil and rosewater. Pour into pot.

Honey and rosewater lip salve
(1 small pot)
3 teaspoons clear honey
1 teaspoon rosewater

Mix ingredients together and just scoop into a small pot. This salve is very good for chapped lips.

Coconut lip salve
(1 small pot)
2 teaspoons beeswax
2 teaspoons coconut oil
1 teaspoon castor oil

Melt the wax in a double boiler or a heat-resistant bowl over hot water, add the oils and mix thoroughly together. Pour into a small pot to set and use as necessary.

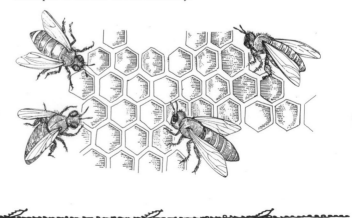

Bath soaks, body creams

The bath soaks and suntan lotions featured on this page can be made simply
with readily available natural ingredients and do not need a full recipe.
Detailed recipes follow on page 85.

Herbal baths

Herbal baths are very quick and easy to prepare, and transform
bath time into a luxuriously aromatic event. The only preparation is to make some simple muslin bags with drawstring tops, so
that they can be filled with the herbs of your choice and tied over
the taps to let the hot water run through them.

All of the following herbs and ingredients have soothing
fragrances. Use one at a time or if preferred, make up
combinations.

Lavender	Camomile	Mint
Rose	Verbena	Yarrow
Rosemary	Pine	Hyssop
Thyme	Balm	Valerian

Herbal bubble baths

To make your own herbal bubble bath, make a 300ml (½ pt) of a
strong (use 25g [1oz] of herbs) herbal infusion see p.20, and beat
in a capful of commercial, unperfumed bubble bath or shampoo.
Then mix with the running water into the bath.

Bath vinegars and oils

A combination of herbs and vinegar makes a stimulating bath
additive that is excellent for maintaining the acid balance of the
skin. To make a herbal vinegar take 50g (2oz) of a dried herb and
place it in a large wide-topped glass jar. Cover with 1 l (2pts) of
cider vinegar. Seal the jar tightly and shake it well. Keep it for
two weeks, shaking every day, then try a little rubbed on the
wrist to see how herby it smells. Add more herbs if necessary.
When the herb vinegar is ready, strain out the herbs and keep
the jar by the bath. Add a cupful to the bath water. Bath oils
either float on the surface, coating your skin as you get out of the
bath, or disperse in the water and soak into the skin.

Suntan lotions

The lotions should be placed in small wide-topped bottles,
except where stated, and will keep indefinitely.

Simple tanning oils – these can be plant oils just used on their
own.

Coconut oil – a thick white oil that looks solid in the jar but
melts in the heat of the sun.

Olive oil – use it on its own or mix with cider vinegar.

Sesame oil – use alone or mix with equal measures of lanolin.
Melt the two together in a double boiler or in a heat-resistant pan
over hot water.

After-sun lotions (To cool sunburnt skin)

Add enough quantities of the following ingredients to soothe the
afflicted areas.

Mashed strawberries

Grated carrot – apply as a poultice (gauze side against the skin)

Cucumber pulp

Bicarbonate of soda – add a cup to a tepid bath

Cider vinegar Make a solution of 1 part vinegar to 3 parts water
and wring out a flannel in the mixture. Apply to sunburnt areas.

Yoghurt Smooth on with cotton wool and leave for half an hour,
splash off.

Witch hazel Soak pads of cotton wool and apply as a compress.

Potato slices Wipe over the skin.

Buttermilk Soak pads of cotton wool in the buttermilk and apply
as a compress.

Cold tea – soak pads of cotton wool in the cold tea and apply as
a compress.

Gin Use the same method as for cold tea.

Camomile or comfrey infusion, Apply cold in compresses.

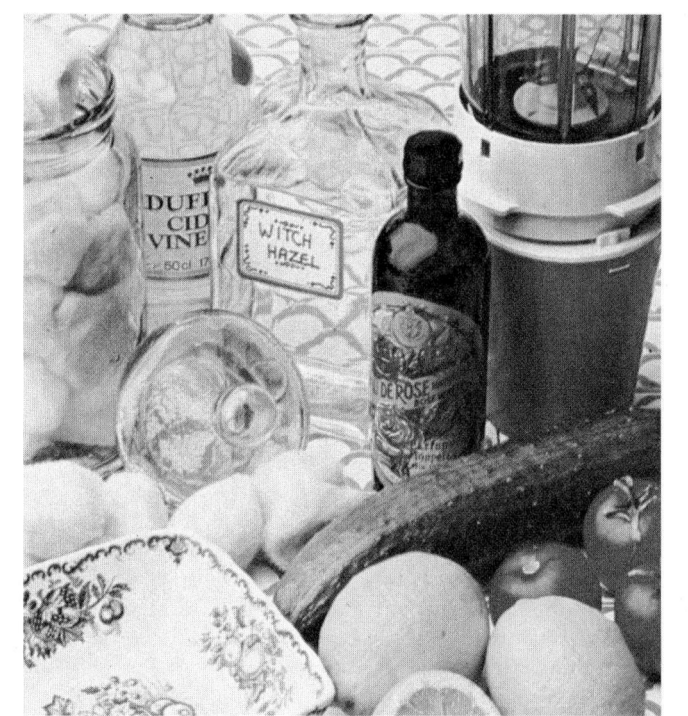

Floating bath oil

(1 application)
2 tablespoons oil such as almond, sunflower, olive, safflower.
5 drops essential oil such as lavender, geranium, sandalwood,
peppermint.

Mix the two oils together and add to the bath water. As you lie in the bath scoop up oil and massage it into your skin.

Honey and milk bath oil

(1 large bottle)
2 eggs
6 tablespoons olive oil
6 tablespoons sunflower oil
1 teaspoon honey
3 teaspoons mild shampoo
6 tablespoons milk
3 tablespoons vodka
few drops perfume oil

Beat the eggs and oils together, then beat in the honey. Continue beating hard while you add the shampoo, milk and vodka. Add drops of the perfume oil to add fragrance. Pour into a large bottle and keep chilled. This is a dispersing bath oil.

Lanolin body oil

(1 medium bottle)
4 tablespoons lanolin
2 tablespoons olive oil
Few drops geranium oil

Melt the lanolin in a double boiler or in a heat-resistant bowl over hot water and stir in the olive oil. Remove from heat. When the mixture is cool add the geranium oil or any other of your choice for fragrance and pour into bottle.

Mixed body oil

(1 medium bottle)
6 tablespoons almond oil
3 tablespoons sunflower oil
3 tablespoons olive oil
3 tablespoons safflower oil
few drops perfume oil

Stir the oils together and add the perfume oil – cinnamon or sandalwood are very good and camphor oil is very warming for tired muscles. Pour into bottle. Massage into the skin after a bath until all the oil is absorbed.

Coconut and sesame body oil

(1 medium bottle)
4 tablespoons coconut oil
4 tablespoons sesame oil
Few drops orange blossom oil

Melt the coconut oil in a double boiler or in a heat-resistant pan over hot water and beat in the sesame oil. Take off heat and when cool add the orange blossom oil and bottle. Again massage into the skin after a bath.

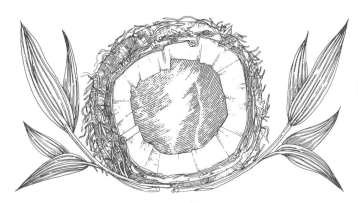

Avocado and wheatgerm body oil

(1 medium bottle)
4 tablespoons avocado oil
4 tablespoons wheatgerm oil
Few drops sandalwood oil

Mix all the oils together and put in a bottle. This oil is very pleasant to use and when massaged into the skin exudes a lovely fragrance. This is particularly good to use after a hard exercising session.

Silky body lotion

(1 medium bottle)
1½ tablespoons soapflakes
6 tablespoons water
2 teaspoons glycerine
4 teaspoons almond oil
1 teaspoon witch hazel
Few drops perfume oil

Dissolve the soapflakes in warm water then remove from the heat and add the glycerine, almond oil and witch hazel. Stir well until cool, then add the perfume oil and bottle. This recipe makes a very pleasant, fluid cream that leaves the skin feeling as soft as silk.

Lavender body lotion
(1 medium bottle)
1 teaspoon borax
6 tablespoons lavender water
4 tablespoons almond oil
Few drops lavender oil

Dissolve the borax in the warmed lavender water then beat in the almond and lavender oils and when cool, put in a bottle. Shake the lotion well before use and massage into the body.

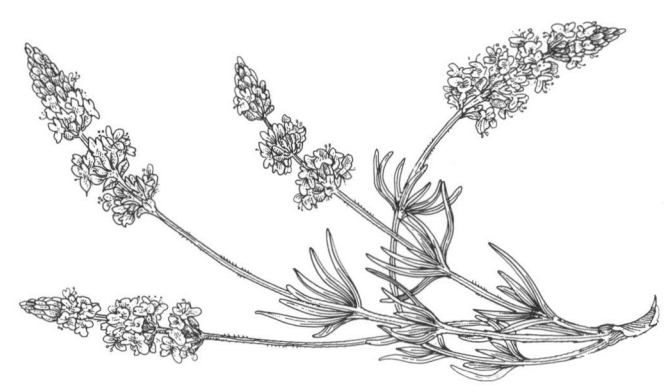

Honey and orange flower body lotion
(1 medium bottle)
2 tablespoons almond oil
2 tablespoons wheatgerm oil
1 tablespoon clear honey
½ teaspoon borax
4 tablespoons orange flower water
Few drops bergamot oil

Mix the oils and honey together. Dissolve the borax in the warmed orange flower water add the perfume oil and whisk all the ingredients together to form a lotion. Bottle, and use as required.

Apricot breast-firming cream
(1 small pot)
1 tablespoon lanolin
1 tablespoon cocoa butter
2 tablespoons apricot oil
1 tablespoon rosewater
½ teaspoon borax

Melt the lanolin and butter in a double boiler or in a heat-resistant pan over hot water, then stir in the apricot oil and remove from heat. Dissolve the borax in the rosewater, then beat all the ingredients together to make a cream. Keep in a small pot.

Breast-firming oil
(1 small pot)
2 tablespoons almond oil
2 tablespoons wheatgerm oil

Blend the almond and wheatgerm oils together to make a quick and simple oil mixture, which should be massaged into the breasts gently, but with rapid upward motions. Use the oil regularly.

Ivy cellulite cream
(1 small pot)
4 tablespoons of strong ivy decoction (see p.20)
2 teaspoons beeswax
1 teaspoon emulsifying wax
4 teaspoons almond oil
Few drops tincture of benzoin

Make a strong decoction of fresh ivy leaves by boiling 2 handfuls in 600ml (1pt) of purified water. Melt the waxes in a double boiler or in a heat-resistant bowl over hot water and stir in the oil. Take from the heat and beat in 4 tablespoons of the ivy decoction, then add the benzoin. Put into a pot and label. Massage this cream into areas of cellulite, on the thighs, for example with a strong kneading action. This will make the skin really tingle as ivy helps to stimulate the blood flow. Use the cream regularly to notice a difference.

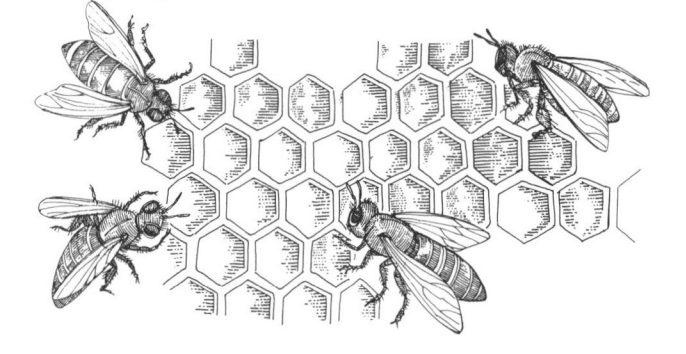

Sesame suntan oil
(1 small bottle)
2 tablespoons lanolin
4 tablespoons sesame oil
6 tablespoons rosewater
1 teaspoon cider vinegar

Melt the lanolin in a double boiler or a heat-resistant bowl over hot water and add the oil. Take off heat and then add the rosewater and vinegar, beating hard to make a lotion. Bottle, and use as required when sunbathing.

Cocoa butter tanning oil

(1 small bottle)

3 tablespoons cocoa butter
3 tablespoons olive oil
3 drops of bergamot oil

Melt the cocoa butter in a double boiler or in a heat-resistant bowl over hot water, stir in the oils. Remove from the heat, leave to cool and bottle. The bergamot oil smells delicious.

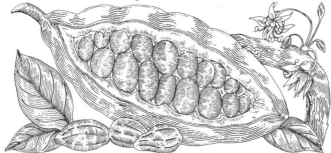

Tea suntan lotion

(1 small bottle)

3 tablespoons coconut oil
3 tablespoons cocoa butter
3 tablespoons olive oil
300ml (½ pt) strong Indian tea

Melt the coconut oil and butter in a double boiler or in a heat-resistant bowl over hot water, then add the olive oil. Remove from the heat and whisk in the tea. Whisk again at regular intervals until completely cool. Bottle and use lavishly. Shake well before use.

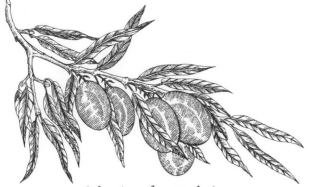

Calamine after-sun lotion

(1 small bottle)

5 teaspoons calamine
6 tablespoons water
2 teaspoons glycerine

Whisk the ingredients together and bottle. Shake before use.

Honey and egg after-sun lotion

(1 application)

1 egg white
1 teaspoon clear honey
1 teaspoon witch hazel

Whisk all the ingredients together and apply gently to afflicted areas for cooling relief.

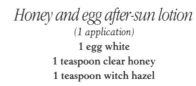

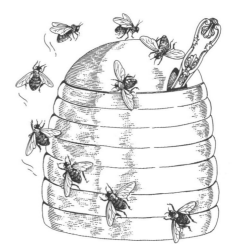

Iodine sunburn oil

(1 small bottle)

6 tablespoons olive oil
3 tablespoons cider vinegar
½ teaspoon iodine
few drops lavender oil

Mix all the ingredients together and bottle. Massage the oily mixture gently into the skin to relieve the burning sensation.

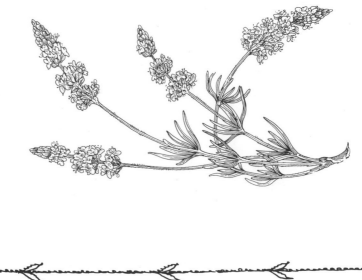

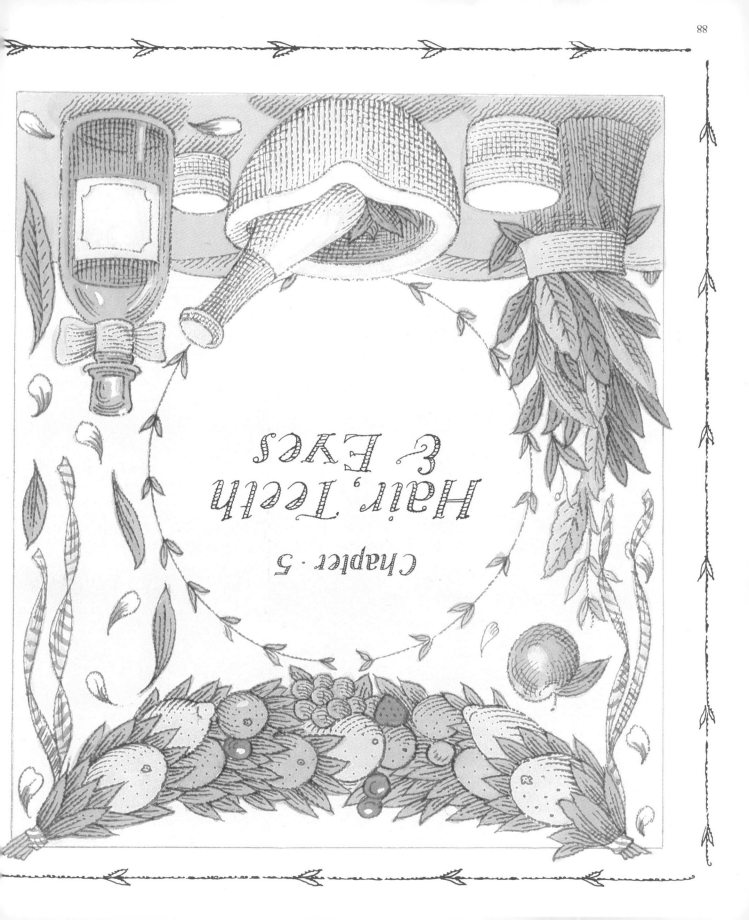

Chapter · 5

Hair, Teeth & Eyes

Hair

Thick, shiny, attractively coloured hair can transform a plain woman into a beauty – no wonder hair is considered a crowning glory. Lucky girls naturally have thick and lustrous locks, but most of us have to contend with hair that is not as full, glossy and manageable as we would like. The first step, in transforming the hair you have into hair to be proud of, is to come to terms with its natural limitations, then boost its appearance with good hair cuts, regular washing, conditioning and perhaps colouring. Like your skin, your hair reflects your general state of health, so it goes without saying that healthy habits give your hair the best possible foundation for growth. Understanding your hair's basic structure will help you to care for it in the right way, and deal with any problems that may occur.

The average scalp has roughly 100,000 hair follicles, five out of six of which have growing hairs at any one time, the sixth goes through a resting phase which will last between two and three months. Each hair has a three to five year growing cycle before it falls out. Hairs on the scalp grow at an average rate of 0.4mm a day (about 1cm (½in) a month). New hair cells are formed in the base of the hair root which is situated in the deepest part of the hair follicle. Just like skin, hair grows as a result of the continuous process of new cells forming, maturing and dying – moving upwards as they do so. Sebaceous glands in the scalp feed each hair shaft with oil to protect it and keep the cells smooth and supple.

The part of your hair that is visible outside the scalp is called the hair shaft, and is composed of three layers. The outer layer is a protective cuticle which is made up of hard, transparent overlapping keratin (a form of protein) scales. If these scales are lying flat, the hair will have a smooth, shiny appearance. But if they are ruffled up, as is the case with dry, damaged hair, the overall appearance of your hair will be dull and fuzzy. Keeping moisture in this outer layer of the hair shaft is fundamental to healthy hair.

Inside the cuticle is the cortex, which consists of tightly intertwined protein fibres in amino-acid chains. These fibres give the hair its strength and elasticity. The cortex also contains the pigment cells that give hair its colour. If this part of the hair becomes too dry, the hair shaft will split.

Inside the cortex is the medulla which is made up of a spongy substance resembling bone marrow. This is connected to the hair root in the follicle.

How hair grows

Hair grows faster in summer than in winter because growth is stimulated by warmth, but it does not grow indefinitely. This growth phase varies from person to person – some people have hair that will only grow for two years, others have hair that will grow for as many as seven years – which means waist length hair. If your hair has a relatively short growth cycle there is nothing you can do to make it grow longer than shoulder length, so it would

A cross-section through a tiny area of the scalp, magnified many times shows how each individual hair grows out of its follicle. New hair cells are formed in the base of each follicle, fed by the blood supply. Near the surface of the skin is a sebaceous gland which feeds the emerging hair with oil to keep it supple.

Sebaceous gland

Medulla

Cortex

Cuticle

be futile trying. When the growth phase of a hair ends, the hair follicle enters a resting phase for a few months. The old hair stops growing and remains in the follicle until a new hair starts to grow up from underneath, so pushing the old hair out. These hairs fall out in the region of 20 to a 100 each day, so do not be alarmed to see hair in the brush or comb.

Your natural hair colour and texture

All the characteristics of your hair, such as the thickness, curliness, dryness and colour are hereditary. All the hair follicles you will ever have are present at birth, and follicles that die never produce another hair. This is why natural male baldness is irreversible. Illness and emotional stress can also cause hair to fall out, but as long as the follicle is still alive it will produce a new hair.

The colour of your hair is determined genetically by the quantity of melanin in the cortex. If you have one dark-haired parent and one with fair hair you are more likely to be dark, as the genes for dark and curly hair dominate those for blonde or straight hair. Mouse-coloured (light brown) hair is the most common hair colour among caucasians. As you get older, less melanin is produced, and so the hair appears white or grey in colour.

For no known scientific reason, blondes tend to have the most hairs but they are finer, while redheads have the least hairs but they tend to be thicker. The curl in your hair or the lack of it depends on the shape of the cells as they leave the follicle.

The only way to permanently change your hair's natural appearance is by using an artificial colourant or a perm, both of which chemically transform the basic structure of the hair. These processes penetrate right through to the cortex and unravel the spiral structure of the fibres, then re-set them in a new form. The result of such harsh treatment can be porous, weak and broken hair. Luckily any abuse inflicted on the visible hair does not affect the hair under the scalp which will grow in a healthy way and be undamaged. It is much wiser to treat your hair with gentle respect, and colour it with herbal dyes which merely stain the outer cuticle. If you long for curls, forget chemical perms which can look tired and dry after a few weeks. Experiment with temporary hair sets such as those achieved by using rag rollers. These curl the hair gently but firmly, and look attractive enough to be worn as hair decorations!

Learning to identify the individual characteristics of your hair will enable you to choose the treatments that will make it look its best. Identifying your hair type is the first step to total hair health.

Your hair type

Normal hair is neither too greasy nor too dry, and when clean looks shiny and smooth. It may be straight or curly but it is easy to manage.
To treat: wash every three to five days, condition every other wash.

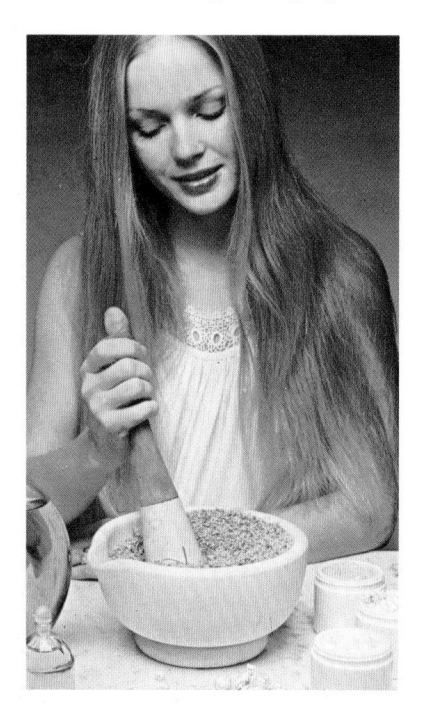

An infusion of camomile flowers makes a gentle lightener for naturally blond hair. You can make a paste to leave on the hair for deeper colouring effects, or just use a camomile rinse after every hair wash to add subtle, golden highlights.

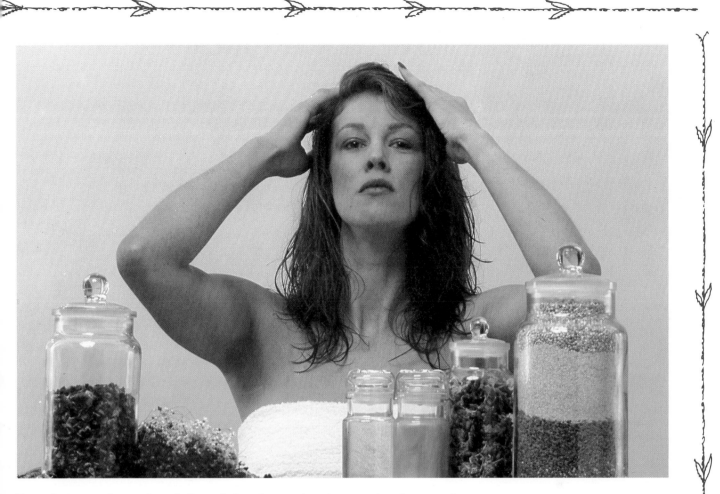

Dry hair tends to be dull and brittle, and splits easily. It may be accompanied by a dry, flaky scalp. This is because too few sebaceous glands are feeding the hair shaft with oil, leaving the hair dry and fragile. This hair type needs a lot of attention.

To treat: shampoo every five to seven days, using a very mild shampoo. A shampoo with added oil will treat your hair gently, but it is wiser to add oil in rich conditioners afterwards. Condition after every wash with one of the rich oily conditioners in the recipe section, and treat your hair occasionally to an extra-deep conditioning hair pack. Perming is definitely not for you, and you should also avoid heated rollers and back-combing. On the plus side, dry hair often has a lot of body and you can have a really full head of hair which is easier to style than oily hair. If the hair is fine, colour can add the illusion of fullness if applied in gentle highlights. A vegetable or herbal tint will colour dry hair gently while protecting the outer cuticle from damage.

Oily hair results from over-generous sebaceous glands, which constantly secrete oil down the hair shafts making the hair oily and lank. It is often joined by dandruff as the excess oil on the scalp slows down the shedding of dead cells, which then build up on the scalp under the hair.

Many herbs are very beneficial to the scalp, fighting dandruff and drying up excess oil. You can add an infusion of your chosen herb to a mild shampoo, or use afterwards as a hair rinse.

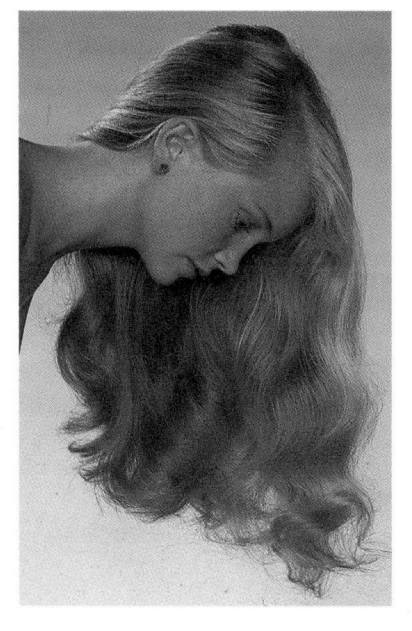

Shiny hair depends on a healthy scalp, and careful attention to washing, conditioning and brushing. Your hair reflects your general state of health, too, so make sure you eat a nutritious diet and get plenty of exercise. Avoid harsh, chemical treatments, and use the natural powers of herbs and flowers to colour and condition your hair.

To treat: wash the hair every day or every other day with a very mild herbal shampoo. Do not be tempted to use strong 'drying' shampoos as these strip away too much oil, leaving you with oily roots and over-dried ends. The bonus with oily hair is that it has a wonderful shine when clean, and has no need for conditioning. Similarly avoid commercial anti-dandruff shampoos as these contain chemicals which are much too harsh for the tender scalp. A natural herbal rinse makes a better solution. If the ends of the hair look dry condition them only. Oily hair is the only hair type that can regularly stand up to mild perming and bleaching, because the drying action of both processes fights the natural greasiness.

Guidelines for healthy hair

• **Take good care** of your scalp as this is where problems often begin. A dry red itchy scalp suggests an allergy to some harsh chemical product, while a pale scalp with a powdery residue could mean dryness due to poor circulation, and insufficient oxygen and essential nutrients reaching the hair follicles. Any unusual, irritating scalp condition should be investigated by a doctor or trichologist. Keep your scalp in tip-top condition by giving it an all over massage when you wash your hair, or when applying a deep-treatment conditioner. When the hair is wet, start at the back of the hair-line with the pads of all ten fingers pressing against the scalp. Work all over the head from back to front actually moving the scalp with a circular motion. This also helps to relax tension, while encouraging the flow of blood.

• **Protect your hair** from strong sunlight and salt water. Hair burns just like skin, and salt water really dries it out. Either wear a protective covering or slick your hair back with a protective oil or conditioner while swimming or sunbathing. (See the relevant recipes).

• **Watch your diet** and general health, both of which affect your hair by slowing the flow of blood to the scalp tissues. A good balanced diet, regular exercise and avoiding stress all help to boost healthy hair growth.

• **Hormones can** dramatically affect your hair. During pregnancy the high level of oestrogen in the body causes hair to grow thick and glossy, as it is oestrogen that stimulates hair growth. Soon after childbirth hair returns to normal, and the resulting hair loss causes many women to think they are losing too much hair. The male sex hormone testosterone is responsible for triggering baldness in men, as a surplus of it destroys hair follicles. It is often said, and it is not entirely untrue, that the balder the man, the more virile! With the onset of the menopause oestrogen production in women falls, and in some cases, can lead to thinning hair, dryness and scalp problems.

• **It is important** not to disturb the hair's natural acid balance, which is also described as the 'pH' balance. A shampoo should be acid enough not to disturb this balance, and the milder the shampoo the better. Too frequent washing with alkaline products is very hard on the hair. Commercial shampoos contain detergent rather than soap, as the latter forms a scum in

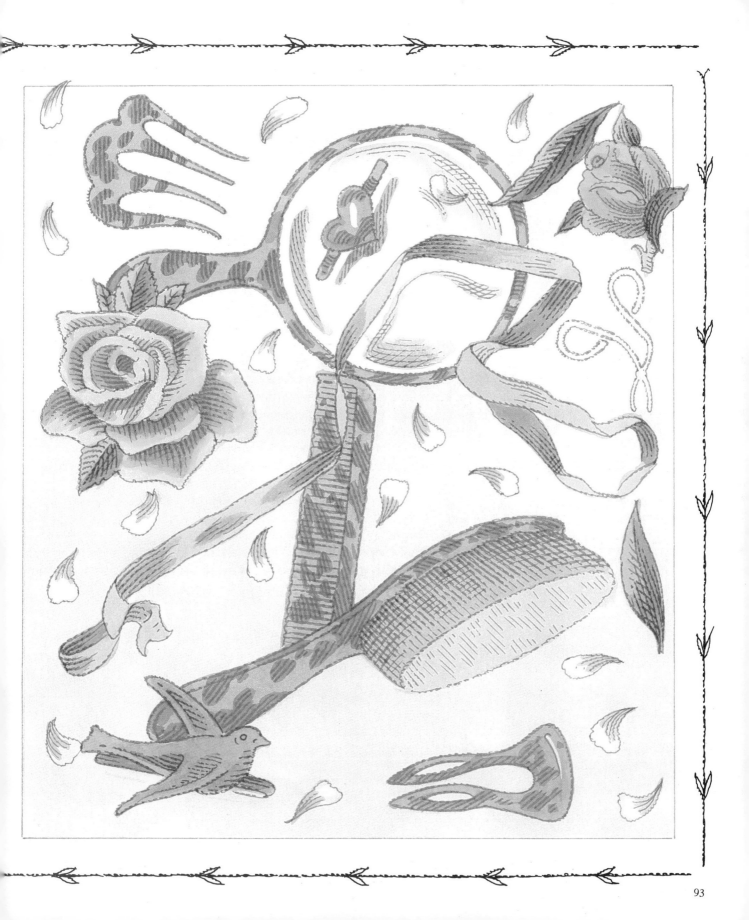

Right: Always wash hair thoroughly in a mild herbal shampoo. Using an acid hair rinse afterwards helps to impart a shine to the hair.

hard water. Some detergents are milder than others, and more diluted with water in a shampoo. The other ingredients in commercial shampoos are perfume, colouring agents, and pearlizers to make the product look pretty. If you do not want to make your own shampoos from scratch, the next best option is to buy the mildest shampoo you can find, such as a baby shampoo, and add a herbal infusion of your choice. Adding oils to shampoos can also give a gentler lather with less risk of stripping away the hair's natural oils, but they will not do such a thorough job of cleansing, and it is better to add oil in your conditioner afterwards, so a fine coating is left on the hair.

Rinsing your hair after shampooing with an acid rinse, containing cider vinegar or lemon, helps to restore the acid mantle to the hair.

Occasional protein packs are good for all hair types, but especially damaged hair, as they strengthen and protect the cuticle. Choose one from the recipe section, and leave it on your hair for 20 minutes or more.

● **When deciding to** change the colour of your hair, take the rest of your skin colouring into account. Dramatic colour changes rarely suit anyone, and it makes more sense, both for your appearance and the health of your hair, to use only herbal tints. Plants and flowers can provide colour changes that vary from the subtle to the vivid, and as they only stain the outer cuticle they will gradually fade out. Experiment to find the one that suits you best, and make stronger infusions for more dramatic results. Henna, which is obtained from the lawsonia plant, provides the strongest red shades, while rhubarb root gives golden tones. Marigold and saffron make hair more golden, while camomile is a gentle lightener for blonde or mousey hair. Privet, sage and walnut leaves can all darken the hair. The mildest bleach of all is lemon juice. Using herbal colourants means you can actually help, not harm your hair while getting the impact of new colour.

1 Hair needs very gentle treatment after shampooing. Squeeze excess moisture from the hair with a towel – do not rub it as this will cause tangles.

2 Wet hair stretches and breaks easily so comb it gently with a wide-toothed comb.

3 When blow-drying your hair, take care not to over-heat the hair by keeping the dryer at least 12cm (6in) from your hair and keep the air stream moving.

● **Brush and comb** your hair gently at all times. Use only bristle brushes, or plastic ones with rounded quills. Never brush your hair when wet, but comb it gently with a wide-toothed comb, as this will prevent stretching and breaking the strands.

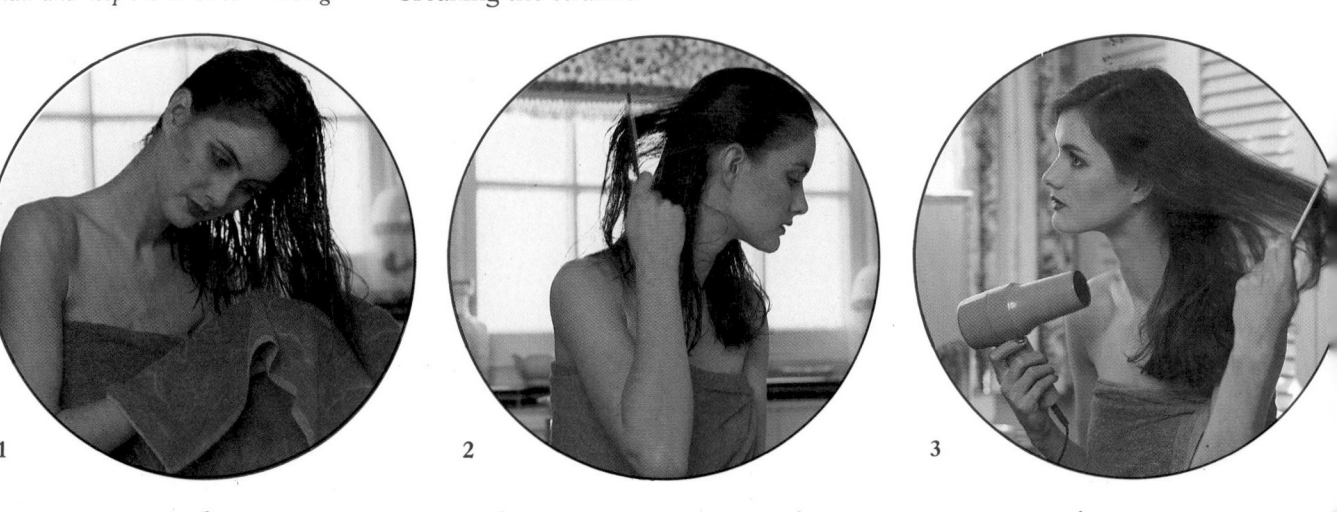

1 2 3

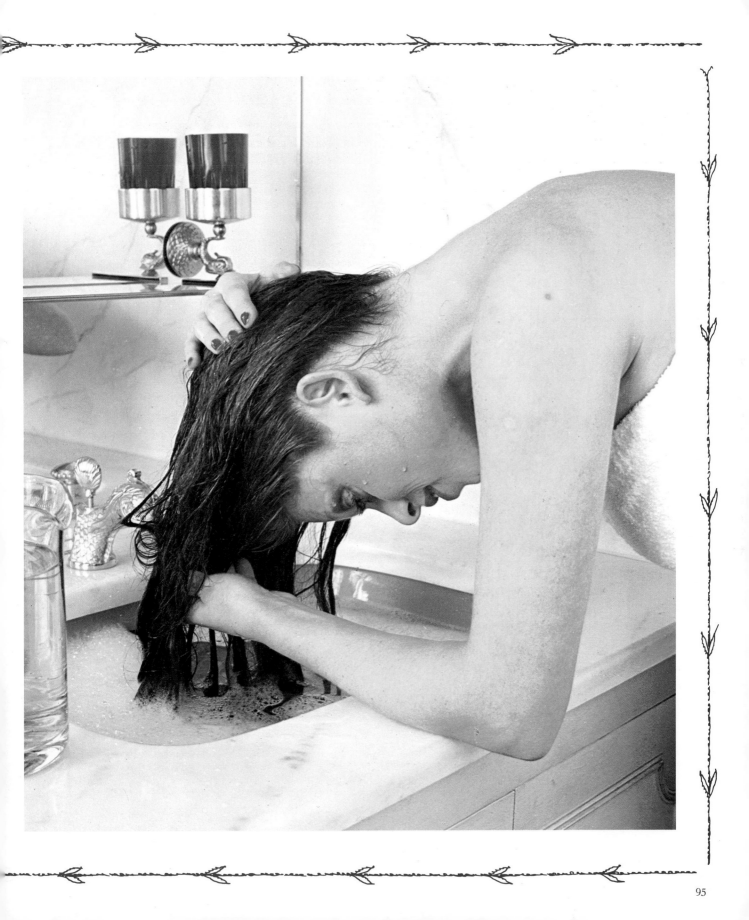

Shampoos, rinses, conditioners and colourants

The shampoo rinses and colourants on this page can be made simply with readily available natural ingredients and do not need a full recipe. Detailed recipes follow on page 97.

Hair shampoos

The simplest way to make a herbal shampoo is to add 2 or 3 tablespoons of a strong (50g [½oz] of the herb to 150ml [¼pt] of purified water) herbal infusion (see page 20) or listed ingredient to a mild baby shampoo. Choose one from the following, according to your hair type.

Oily hair
Lemon juice, add 4 tablespoons to shampoo
Lavender infusion
Marigold infusion
Yarrow infusion
Witch hazel, add 2 tablespoons to shampoo

Normal or dry hair
Comfrey infusion
Marshmallow infusion
Sage infusion
Elderflowers infusion
Lecithin, add 3 tablespoons to shampoo
Egg yolks, (beaten) add two to shampoo

Dandruff
Rosemary infusion
Nettle infusion
Thyme infusion
Parsley infusion

Hair rinses

A final rinse with a natural ingredient enhances the colour of your hair, restores the acid balance and encourages shine. Try any of the following to find out which one particularly suits your hair type.
Cider vinegar Suits all hair types. Add a few drops to the final rinsing water.
Nettle, sage or parsley Improves all hair colours and adds body.
Elderflower For normal to dry hair
Lavender For oily hair
Rosemary For dandruff
Comfrey For sensitive scalps

Make a strong (use 50g) [2oz] of the herb) infusion (see p. 20) of one of the above herbs and add to final rinse.

Mix the herbal infusion with cider vinegar or lemon juice for extra strength.

Hair colourants

Several herbs are renowned for their abilities to add shine and to lighten, darken or add a red tint to the hair. They can be used as straightforward rinses or pastes.

To make a rinse, you will need a strong infusion of your chosen herb (see list) in the ratio of 4 tablespoons of the herb to 600ml (1pt) of purified water, and pour it over the hair as a final rinse. This will impart soft highlights.

For Fair Hair
Camomile infusion (mild)
Rhubarb root (decoction – see page 20)
Mullein infusion
Lemon (dilute the juice of ½ lemon in water). For stronger highlights rub ½ a lemon onto hair before going in the sun.

For Red Hair
Marigold infusion
Saffron infusion
Red oak bark infusion
Ginger root (decoction – see page 20)

For Dark Hair
Walnut leaves infusion
Rosemary infusion
Cloves infusion
Privet infusion

For Grey Hair
Sage infusion
Elderberry infusion

Colouring pastes
These give a stronger result than rinses, and can be left on the hair for as long as you like.

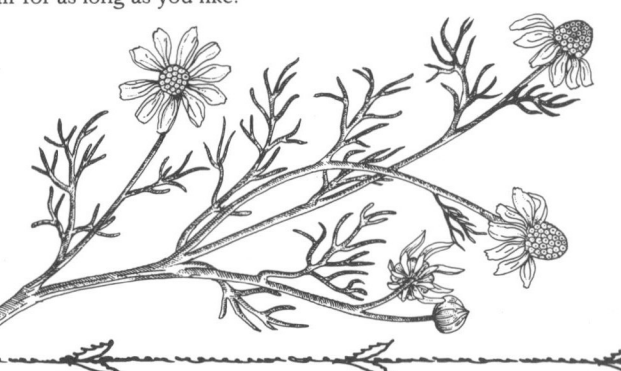

Herbal Castile soap shampoos
(1 medium bottle)
25g (1oz) of chosen herb for your hair type (see p. 96)
600ml (1pt) water
25g (1oz) grated soap
Few drops of essential oil for perfume

Make an infusion (see p. 20) of the herb and allow it to strengthen over night. Strain through coffee filter paper and pour it in a saucepan. Add the soap and heat gently until the soap melts. Allow to cool and add the perfume oil. Pour into a bottle. In cold weather the soap content may start to solidify, so simply warm the bottle gently before use.

Castile or plain white unperfumed soap is more gentle on the hair than detergent-based bought shampoo. It will not lather up as much, so you may need to use slightly more of it.

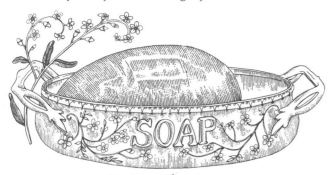

Soapwort shampoos
(1 medium bottle)
15g (½oz) crushed soapwort root, leaves or stems
1l (2pt) water

Make an infusion (see p. 20) of the soapwort root and leave to stand for several hours, shaking the jar from time to time. Strain, and add to this 6 tablespoons of the herbal infusion of your choice suitable for your hair type (see p. 96).

A soapwort infusion makes a naturally soapy liquid. You will need about half a cup of soapwort shampoo to wash your hair, more if it is long.

Orris root dry shampoo
(1 application)
2 tablespoons powdered orris root
2 tablespoons, salt, arrowroot or bicarbonate of soda

Massage powdered orris root into the scalp and brush gently through the hair. Leave for 30 minutes then brush out briskly with a clean brush. Orris root can be mixed with 2 tablespoons of salt, arrowroot or bicarbonate of soda for a similar effect.

Fuller's earth and bran dry shampoo
(1 application)
1 tablespoon fullers' earth powder
2 tablespoons bran

Pound the bran to a fine powder and add the fullers' earth. Massage into the scalp and comb through hair. Brush out after 30 minutes with a bristle brush. Substitute the bran with ground almond meal or oatmeal. Ideal for normal or oily hair.

Flower water dry shampoo
(1 application)
1 pieece of gauze soaked in lavender water)

When hair is very oily, try refreshing it with a piece of gauze soaked in lavender water. Force the gauze over the bristles of your hairbrush and brush until cloth shows the grime. Repeat with fresh gauze (again soaked in lavender water) until hair looks fresher. Use for normal or oily hair but for dry hair, substitute rosewater as it is more effective.

Honey and egg conditioner
(pre-conditioner)
(1-2 applications)
1 teaspoon honey
2 teaspoons safflower, olive or almond oil
1 egg

Combine honey and oil together, then blend in the egg. Massage into the hair and comb through. Wrap head in a warm towel or cover with a shower cap and leave for 30 minutes. Then shampoo in the normal way. This conditioner is particularly good for split ends.

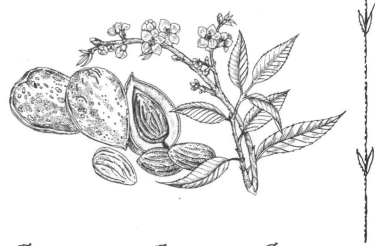

Avocado and egg conditioner
(pre-shampoo)
(1-2 applications)
2 tablespoons avocado oil
1 tablespoon castor oil
1 egg

Combine the oils and blend in the egg, then use as described in the recipe for Honey and egg conditioner on page 97.

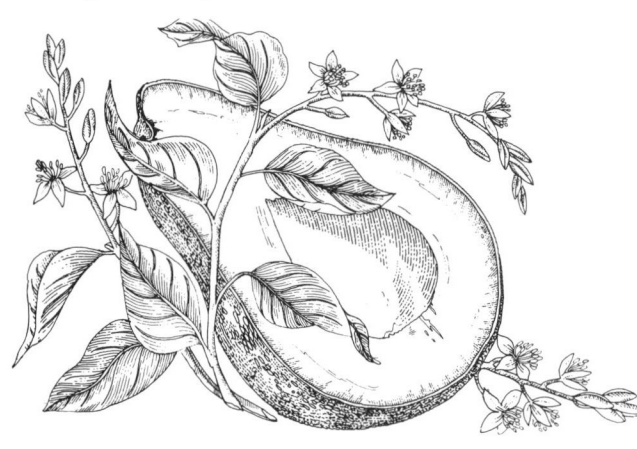

Mayonnaise conditioner
(pre-shampoo)
(1-2 applications)
2 tablespoons olive oil
2 tablespoons cider vinegar
2 eggs

Mix all the ingredients together whisking firmly. Massage into the hair and comb through. Wrap head in a warm towel or cover with a shower cap and leave for 30 minutes. Then shampoo in the normal way.

Avocado conditioner
(after-shampoo)
(1-2 applications)
½ ripe avocado peeled and mashed
1 teaspoon avocado oil
1 egg yolk

Whisk ingredients together then massage into the hair. Leave for a few minutes then rinse with lots of warm water. This light conditioner is ideal for dry hair.

Yoghurt conditioner
(after-shampoo)
(1-2 applications)
5 tablespoons natural yoghurt
1 egg

Whisk the yoghurt and the egg together and massage well into the scalp. Leave for a few minutes then rinse out thoroughly. This conditioner is good for hair that tends to be oily and fly-away.

Brandy Conditioner
(after-shampoo)
(1-2 applications)
2 tablespoons brandy
1 egg

Whisk together the brandy and egg and massage well into the scalp, then wash off after ten minutes. This conditioner makes oily hair more manageable.

Cocoa butter conditioner
(For use in the sun)
(1-2 applications)
1 tablespoon cocoa butter
1 tablespoon lanolin
4 tablespoons olive, safflower or almond oil

Melt all three ingredients in a double boiler and beat together when melted. Add 1 tablespoon of water to 3 tablespoons of the mixture before applying to hair. Shampoo out after about 3 hours of sunbathing.

Coconut oil conditioner
(For use in the sun)
(1-2 applications)
1 tablespoon coconut oil
3 tablespoons castor oil

Melt the two oils together in a double boiler. Apply to scalp and massage well in while still warm. Shampoo out after 3 hours of sunbathing.

Camomile paste (for fair hair)
(1 application)
50g (2oz) camomile
300ml (½pt) purified water
6 tablespoons kaolin powder

Make a very strong infusion of the herb and water, leave over night then strain through a sieve. Add the kaolin powder to make a paste and massage into the hair. Leave as long as you like, or let it dry in the sun, then rinse off with warm water.

Rhubarb root paste (for brown hair)
(1 application)
300ml (½pt) strong rhubarb root decoction (see p. 20)
6 tablespoons kaolin powder
1 egg yolk
1 teaspoon cider vinegar

Add enough of the decoction to the kaolin powder to make a paste, then stir in the egg and vinegar. Leave on the hair for 30-45 minutes, then rinse off in warm water.

Mullein and lemon paste (for golden hair)
(1 application)
300ml (½pt) mullein infusion (see p. 20)
Juice of a lemon
6 tablespoons kaolin powder

Add the lemon juice to the infusion and stir enough of the infusion in the kaolin powder to make a paste. Leave on the hair for 30-45 minutes, then rinse off in warm water.

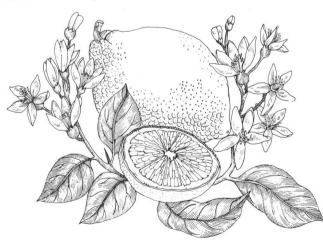

Henna and camomile paste (for light red hair)
(1 application)
6 tablespoons henna powder
300ml (½pt) camomile infusion (see p. 20)
1 teaspoon vinegar or lemon juice

Put the henna powder in a bowl and add enough of the camomile infusion and vinegar or lemon juice to make a paste. Apply the paste to the hair. Keep warm for 30 to 45 minutes then rinse off. Adding more henna will make a stronger colour.

Henna and beetroot paste (for plum red hair)
(1 application)
1 beetroot
6 tablespoons henna powder

Boil the beetroot in water to get a strong decoction (see p. 20). Pour enough over the henna powder to get a smooth paste and massage into the hair. Leave for 30-45 minutes and rinse out. For a really adventurous colour leave the paste for a longer time on the head.

Walnut paste (to darken brown hair)
(1 application)
6 tablespoons green walnut skins
2 tablespoons alum powder
6 tablespoons orange flower water

Chop the walnut skins as finely as possible and mix in the alum powder. Add enough orange flower water to make a paste, then massage into the hair and leave for an hour. Shampoo out.

Sage and tea paste (for grey hair)
(1 application)
2 tablespoons dried sage
1 tablespoon Indian tea
6 tablespoons kaolin powder

Infuse the sage and the tea together in 600ml (1pt) of water. Pour enough over the kaolin to make a paste, and massage into the hair. Leave 30 minutes and rinse out.

Teeth

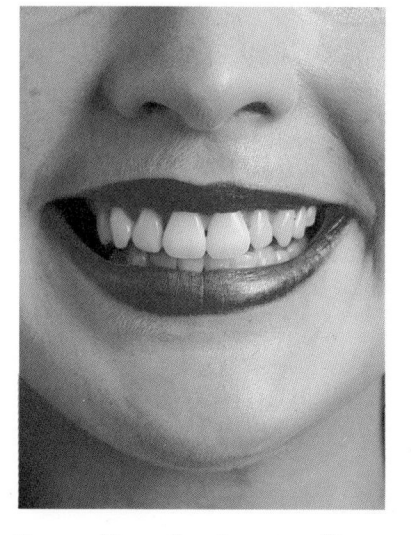

Strong white teeth and sweet-smelling breath depend on careful dental hygiene. Brush with toothpaste twice a day, use dental floss to clean in between each tooth, and visit your dentist for a check-up every six months. There should be no need for fillings if you follow these simple rules.

Your teeth are seen by other people every time you laugh or smile – so it is very important to keep them in the best possible condition. Chipped yellow teeth are unsightly and demoralising, and with today's advanced dental care there is no excuse for a neglected mouth. Some people are lucky enough to have teeth that remain strong and white however little care they are given, but most of us soon suffer from toothache and bleeding gums if we ignore any early warning signs. Save yourself the time and anxiety of frequent visits to the dentist by resolving to take maximum care of your teeth right now. And that means paying attention to hygiene. More teeth are lost through haphazard cleaning than for any other reason. Just a few minutes a day will ensure sparkling teeth and sweet breath.

Your teeth should be evenly coloured but not necessarily gleaming white in order to be healthy. Very white teeth may actually have a softer covering of enamel than yellower teeth. Hard enamel is thin and clear, showing the yellow dentine that is inside each tooth. If your teeth are naturally rather yellow take comfort in the thought that they are probably strong, and as long as they are clean and even in shape, they can look perfectly attractive. Whatever you do resist the temptation to scrub at them with abrasive commercial products designed to remove the stains from teeth. They are not dirty, so abrading them will not do them any good.

Healthy gums are as important as healthy teeth. They should be pale pink and firm, with a matt surface. If they are spongy or red and bleed when you clean your teeth, they need immediate attention. It is a myth that everyone loses their teeth in the end as an inevitable result of the ageing process. An inadequate diet, too much sugar and a lack of hygiene are the main culprits.

Aching teeth and consistently bleeding gums are the signs that something is wrong in your mouth. Toothache usually means you have a cavity that needs filling, and bleeding is often the first sign of gum disease – the major cause of tooth loss.

Plaque – the number one enemy

Plaque is the most common cause of both tooth decay and gum disease. It is a transparent, sticky film that builds up over the surfaces of the teeth if they are not cleaned thoroughly and regularly. Plaque is bacteria which is formed from various substances in the mouth. It gets lodged between the teeth and around the gum margins. Although it is invisible you can feel plaque if you run your tongue over uncleaned teeth – they feel unpleasantly furry. Sugars in the food we eat combine with the bacteria in plaque and acids are produced that attack the tooth enamel and burn tiny holes in it. Left unchecked, these holes can develop into cavities which have to be filled by a dentist in order to save the rest of the tooth. The dentine is attacked first and then the nerve can become eaten away.

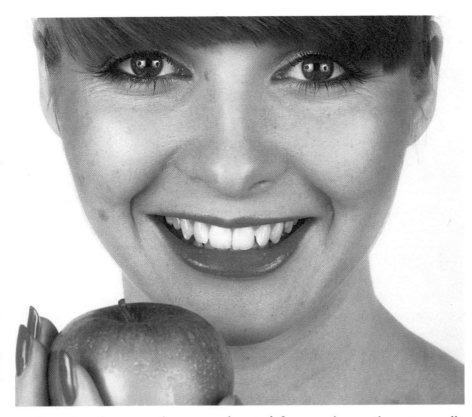

Your teeth are affected by what you eat. Cut right down on sugars which are the prime cause of tooth decay, and try to eat plenty of crunchy fruits such as apples, carrots and celery. A well-balanced diet containing plenty of protein, vitamins and minerals is important for the maintenance of healthy teeth and of gums.

Gum disorders can often go undetected for months, as there is usually little pain. Plaque collects around the area where each tooth meets the gum, and acids attack the gum, causing it to become red and swollen. Soon the gums start to bleed, and if this condition, known as gingivitis, is allowed to continue unchecked, the acids will attack the fibres that hold the tooth in the jaw. The tooth will then become loose and fall out. If plaque is left on the teeth for a long time it starts to harden and has to be removed by a dentist.

Guidelines for healthy teeth

● **The most important** action you can take to ensure strong, evenly-coloured teeth is to keep them clean with regular brushing. This means brushing with toothpaste at least twice a day, followed by the use of dental floss. But do not brush more than three times a day, as over-brushing can wear away the enamel and make teeth more vulnerable to cavities. Use a dry toothbrush and a miminal amount of toothpaste, and brush with short upward movements from gums to teeth edges, both inside and out, paying special attention to the gum margins and the biting surfaces.

Commercial toothpastes contain abrasives, detergents, humectants, binders and flavours. You can make your own toothpastes that are just as effective, but less abrasive and harmful to enamel as some of the commercial ones. The most useful additive in commercial toothpastes is fluoride. This is a mineral which strengthens the surfaces of your teeth, protecting them against decay, so if you are using a herbal toothpaste it would be worthwhile to use also fluoride tablets which are swished around the mouth as they dissolve. Many areas add fluoride to the water supply.

● **If your teeth** are very stained with nicotine or tannin, avoid very abrasive smokers' toothpastes as these are much too harsh on tooth enamel. Use salt or bicarbonate of soda instead, as described in the following recipes.

● **Pick a toothbrush** that has firm, flexible, densely-packed nylon bristles, and a flat surface. Brushes which are too hard are not kind to delicate gum tissue. It is a good idea to have two brushes in use, so that you always have a dry one to work with. Renew your brushes at least every three months, or as soon as they start to fray.

● **Once a day** after brushing, floss your teeth. Dental floss is a fine nylon thread coated with wax which can be slid down or up between each tooth to the gum margin, and then pulled up again removing plaque as it goes. It is a little tricky to get the right knack of flossing to start with, but it soon becomes easy, and should take no longer than two minutes to perform. To use it correctly, take 60cm (2ft) of floss and wind the ends around the middle fingers of each hand. Use your thumbs and index fingers to pull the floss taut, leaving about 10cm (4in) to work with. Gently slide the floss between each tooth, moving from biting edge to gum on the left-hand side of the tooth, rubbing gently as you return it to the edge, then repeat up and down the right-hand side. As the floss becomes frayed wind it along from one finger to the other.

● **Avoid commercial** antiseptic mouthwashes as these are usually much too strong and can upset the natural balance of your mouth. Choose a herbal one from the following recipe section instead, and use whenever you want to ensure sweet-smelling breath. Persistent bad breath is a signal that something is wrong either with the teeth or digestive system, and medical help should be sought. Likewise herbal remedies for toothache can be used as a temporary measure, but only until it is time for your appointment with the dentist.

● **Watch your diet** and make sure you get enough protein which is essential in the formation and maintenance of healthy teeth and gums. Vitamins and minerals are equally important, and lack of calcium (particularly in pregnancy) weakens the tooth enamel. Vitamin C is very helpful in strengthening the tissues. Eat foods that demand a lot of chewing as this increases the saliva production in the mouth, which in turn restores calcium and phosphorus depleted by plaque. Eat plenty of crunchy fruits and vegetables such as apples, carrots and celery. Cut right down on sugar as this combines with plaque to form a substance called dextran which produces the acids that eat away at the teeth.

● **Try to regard** your dentist as a friend and visit him every six months for a check-up. Putting visits off will only involve more visits later!

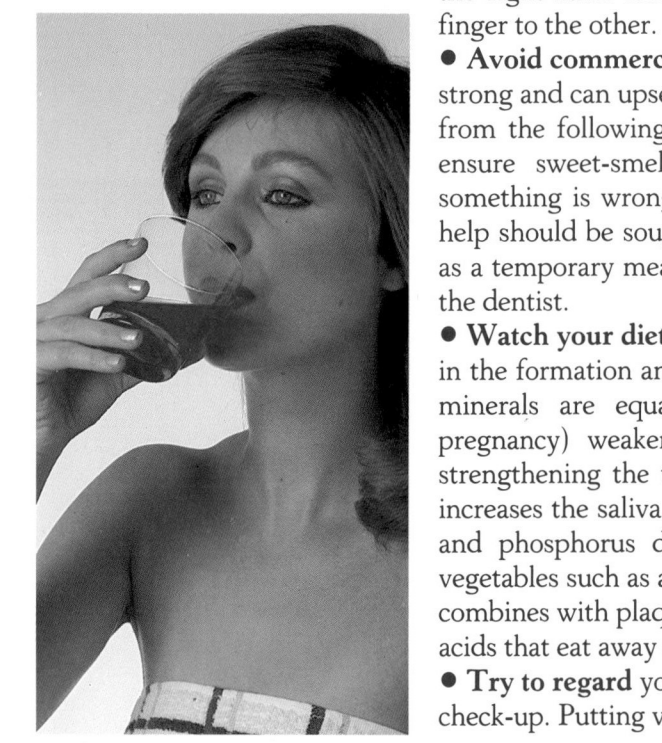

Herbal mouthwashes freshen the breath without upsetting the natural balance of your mouth. Antiseptic mouthwashes can often be too strong and seriously irritate the mouth.

Teeth cleansers and mouthwashes

The teeth cleansers and breath fresheners in the first column on this page can be made simply with natural ingredients and do not need a full recipe. Detailed recipes follow on.

Simple teeth cleansers

The following natural ingredients can used on their own, or with water, to clean teeth. They can be combined with others to make pastes and powders.

Sage Use fresh leaves and rub them over the teeth and gums.
Strawberry Rub slices of the fresh fruit over the teeth to remove stains.
Bicarbonate of soda Sprinkle half a teaspoon on a damp toothbrush to remove stains.
Lemon peel Rub the peel over the teeth to remove brown stains, then rinse with water.
Salt Make a paste with water and dip toothbrush into it.

Simple breath fresheners

Chew fresh leaves of the following herbs to make your breath smell fresher, or make a mild infusion (see page 20, but use only 300ml [½pt] of water to 15g [½oz]).

Parsley
Watercress
Nettle tips
Rose water, gargle with it and spit out
Lavender water, gargle with it and spit out
Cloves, chew them whole or use oil of cloves to rub on gums to ease toothache.
Witch hazel, dilute 1 tablespoon in 6 tablespoons of water, gargle with it and spit out

Salt and sage stain remover
(3-4 applications)
2 tablespoons sea salt
2 tablespoons fresh or dried sage

Pound the two ingredients together with a pestle in a mortar and place the powder in a warm oven. When the mixture has blackened pound it again. Store in an airtight container, and sprinkle on a damp toothbrush. Rinse mouth with water afterwards.

Bicarbonate of soda, salt and peel tooth powder
(3-4 applications)
The dried peel of an orange and/or lemon
2 tablespoons bicarbonate of soda
2 tablespoons sea salt

Grate or pound the orange or lemon peel into powder with a pestle in a mortar, and mix with the other ingredients. Store in an airtight container. Sprinkle a little powder on a damp toothbrush. This powder is good for stained teeth.

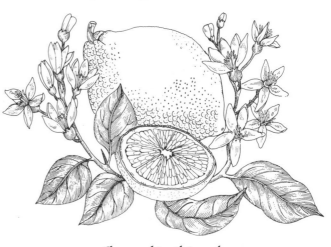

Charcoal tooth powder
(3-4 applications)
2 slices of burnt toast
Few drops of peppermint or clove oil

Pound the toast into powder with a pestle in a mortar, then add the oil for flavour. Store in an airtight container. Sprinkle on a damp toothbrush. Rinse mouth thoroughly after use.

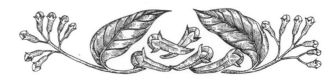

Orris root tooth powder
(3-4 applications)
2 tablespoons orris root
2 tablespoons bicarbonate of soda

Mix the ingredients together. You can also try this recipe with charcoal instead of bicarbonate of soda. Store in an airtight container. Sprinkle the mixture onto a damp toothbrush.

Cinnamon and arrowroot toothpaste

(3-4 applications)

4 tablespoons arrowroot
2 tablespoons ground cinnamon

Store the two ingredients in a an airtight container and mix some when needed with a little water to make a paste. Dip a dry toothbrush into the mixture. This is an ideal toothpaste for sensitive teeth.

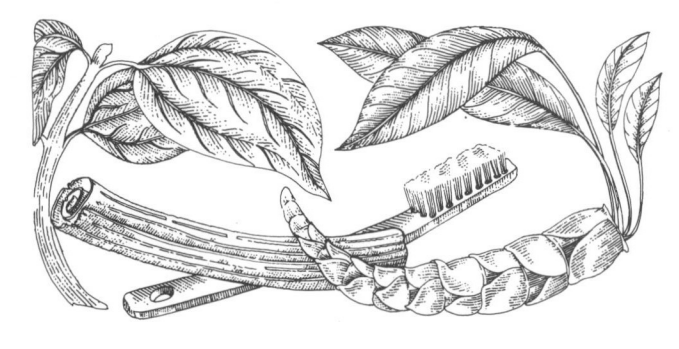

Almond and camphor toothpaste

(1 application)

1 tablespoon ground almonds
1 teaspoon camphor BP
1 teaspoon sea salt
Few drops of clove oil

Pound the dry ingredients together with a pestle in a mortar then add water to make a smooth paste. Stir in the oil. Then dip a dry brush in the mixture.

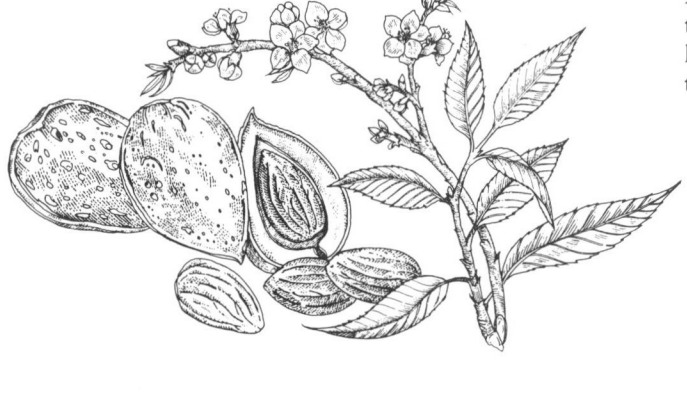

Mint and rosemary mouthwash

(1 application)

½ teaspoon mint
½ teaspoon rosemary
½ teaspoon tincture of myrrh

Make an infusion of the rosemary and mint in 600ml (1pt) of boiling purified water, strain and add the tincture of myrrh. When the mixture is cool, swish it around the mouth and spit out. The mint and rosemary will sweeten the breath while the myrrh acts as a mild antiseptic.

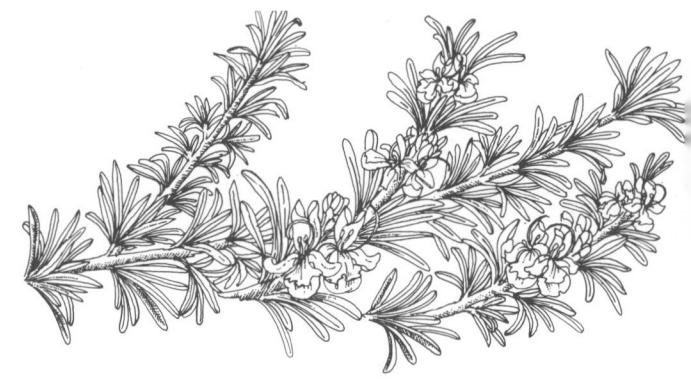

Spicy mouthwash

(1 application)

1 tablespoon ground nutmeg
1 tablespoon ground cloves
½ tablespoon ground caraway seeds
½ tablespoon ground cinnamon
150ml (¼pt) sweet sherry

Pound all the dry ingredients together with a pestle in a mortar, then place in an airtight container and add the sherry. Seal and leave to macerate for a few days. Strain and add a few drops of the sweet-tasting mouthwash to a tumbler of water.

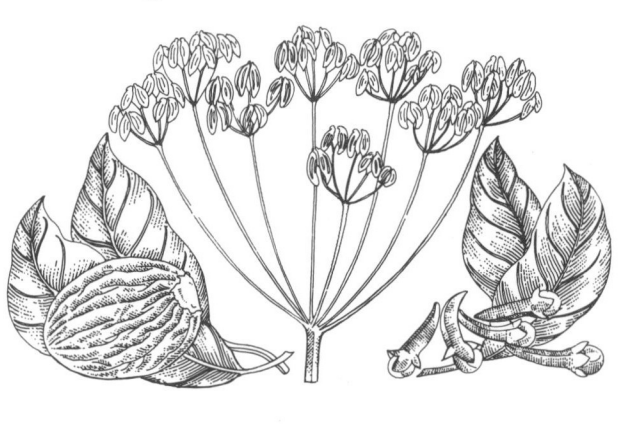

The eyes

Beautiful eyes are supposed to be the most valuable asset a woman can have. Not only do expressive eyes transform a face, they say more about that person's personality and mood than any word or gesture.

Eyes that possess an alluring shape and colour can not be achieved – you have to be born with them, but any eyes that are sparkling and clear can be beautiful. It is not always possible to think wonderful thoughts and gaze warmly upon the world – but you can make sure that your eyes never betray you by looking bloodshot, droopy and tired.

Healthy eyes really shine, with a blue-white tint to the whites of the eyeballs and no hint of redness in the eyes or surrounding eyelids. Eyes do an excellent job of looking after themselves. They keep moist and protected from irritation by a film of fluid spread across the eyeball by the frequent blinking of the eyelids. Eyes have to cope with many irritants such as pollution, smoke, dried-out air as a result of central heating, cold air, wind and eye make-up. Tears from the lacrimal glands deal admirably with all these unwelcome guests by washing them out, while the eyelashes that fringe the eyes try to trap these invaders before they get in. The eyes often over-water if the irritation is persistent and difficult to eject. Interestingly, an excess of emotion, whether you feel happy or sad, has the same effect, causing tears to ooze out of the eyes. Never rub your eyes when this happens as it will make them red and sore. Better to blot them gently with a tissue and try to enjoy the thorough eye-bath your eyes are experiencing! It is the rubbing rather than the tears themselves that leads to red, throbbing eyes after a crying session.

Sometimes tears alone cannot deal with continuous irritation, and eyes need bathing to restore their clarity. The simplest eye-bath of all is a weak solution of salt and water, with a fresh wash for each eye, so that you do not transfer infection from one eye to the other. Infusions of certain herbs and flowers are also famed for their soothing properties. The best known is the aptly named eyebright, which has anti-inflammatory actions.

The area of skin surrounding the eyes is much finer and thinner than on the rest of the face, and it is meagrely supplied with oil glands. The eye area is the first to show lines of ageing and expression, and short of holding your face completely immobile right through your life there is little you can to do prevent *some* lines appearing. But keeping the area well-moisturized with a gentle eye cream can help to minimize wrinkles by protecting the delicate skin from moisture loss. A vegetable oil such as avocado or apricot is ideal for this task. Only apply the barest minimum, pat around the eye with the tip of the finger, never rub. When applying any cosmetic to the eyes, be it cleanser, moisturizer or coloured shadow, try to move the actual eyelid and under-eye skin as little as possible. Stroke shadows on gently, and remove them with the lightest possible touch. Never use too much cream around the eyes as this can cause unattractive puffiness due to the retention of fluid.

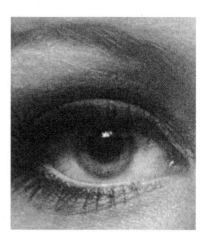

Eyes again reflect your diet and general health. Healthy eyes can be one of the most attractive features in a face. They should really shine and have a blue-white tint to the whites of the eyeballs.

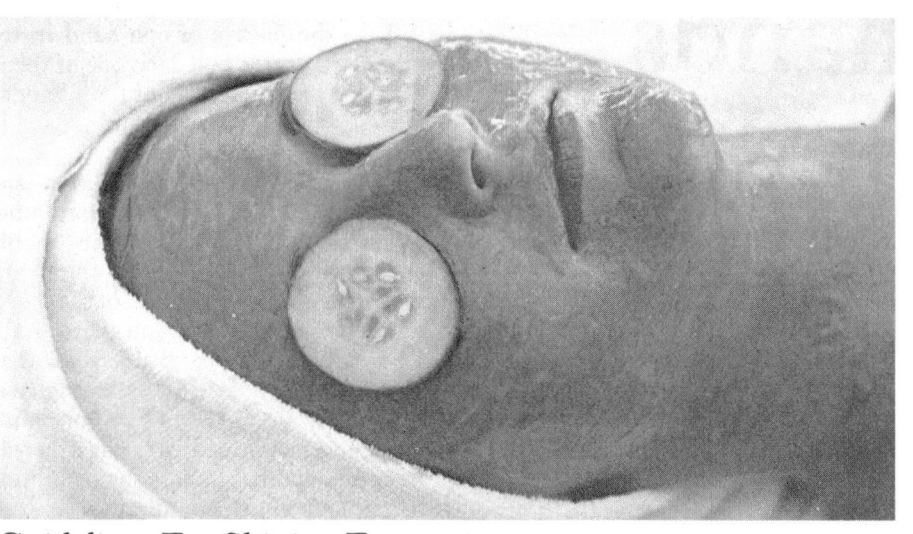

Tired, itchy eyes can be soothed and revived with eyepads. Cucumber slices are particularly cooling and reduce any puffiness or swelling. Relax with eyepads whenever you use a face mask.

Guidelines For Shining Eyes

● **Eyes enjoy the sun** – but only in moderation. Artificial indoor light does not contain the full spectrum of light rays on which eyes thrive, and consequently too much time spent indoors can sap your vitality. Unfiltered sunlight in reasonable amounts revives and strengthens the eyes. Sunglasses can do more harm than good if you wear them continuously, but they are helpful if you are in very bright sunlight for prolonged periods of time, such as when by the sea or when skiing. Eyes burn more easily than skin, so it makes sense to protect them when sunbathing, and wearing sunglasses will stop you squinting which will lead to wrinkles. Choose polarized lenses when by sea or snow, and photochromatic lenses which darken under ultra-violet rays for ordinary wear.

● **Look to your diet**. Good nutrition does more for your eyes than any other factor. A diet rich in vitamins is an all-round beautifier – and the eyes benefit particularly from an eating regime that includes plenty of vitamins A, B and C. This means lots of fresh fruit and vegetables, including carrots. The old wives' tale about carrots helping you to see in the dark has some scientific backing – carrots are rich in Vitamin A. Wheatgerm and yoghurt are also valuable foods. Restrict your intake of alcohol – this dehydrates the eyes and makes them bloodshot.

● **Use cosmetics carefully**. Eye make-up products are especially formulated to treat the eye area gently, but mascara in particular can sting the eyes. Always remove every last trace of eye make-up at night, using a special eye make-up removing lotion. Never sleep in eye make-up, no matter how tired you are, as powders and creams settle into warm skin over night, resulting in red, itchy lids in the morning. Give your eyes a rest from eye make-up for occasional periods.

● **Eyes need exercise**, but too much of the same work can lead to eyestrain. When focussing for long periods on work close by, rest your eyes by looking far into the distance at regular intervals. Exercise the muscles around the eyeball by rotating the eyes. First look up (without moving your head), then look to your right, then carry on moving your eyes round as if looking at all the numbers on a clock face. This exercise really makes the eyes feel wide open and refreshed.

To refresh tired eyes try a trick called palming. Sit with your elbows resting on a table and cover your closed eyes with the palms of your hands. Press gently against the whole area for a couple of minutes. When you take your hands away your vision will be blurry, but it will clear leaving your eyes revived.

● **Massage can put** the sparkle back into tired eyes. Using the tips of the middle fingers, exert gently pressure starting from the bridge of the nose and tap across the eyelids and outwards under the eyes half a dozen times. Then press quite hard on either side of the bridge of the nose close to the inner eye.

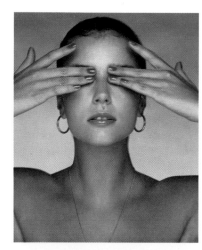

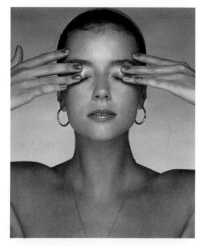

Above and top: Gentle massage can relieve aching eyes. Use the tips of the fingers to stroke gently across the eyelids, working outwards from the bridge of the nose to the temples.

Eye problems and solutions

Puffy eyes can be due to lack of sleep, lack of fresh air, a bad diet, smoky atmosphere, or the condition may be due to a sinus problem such as hay fever. Try a light massage, with a little vegetable oil such as almond oil spread over the cheekbones. Then using the knuckles of your first fingers press firmly outwards from the sides of the nose and under the cheekbones.

A herbal gel patted around the eyes can help to reduce puffiness, and eye pads are cooling and relaxing. There are many varieties for you to try, from raw potato or cucumber slices to pads soaked in herbal infusions. Iced witch hazel is particularly good.

Dark circles under the eyes are often a hereditary trait, caused by thin skin under the eyes revealing the veins close to the surface which appear bluish-black. All you can do in hereditary cases is conceal them with an under-eye concealer cream. But dark circles can also be caused by lack of sleep and poor diet. Drink plenty of water and take part in some outdoor exercise, and try some soothing eyepads.

Bloodshot eyes are most often the result of too little sleep, smoky atmospheres and over-indulgence in alcohol. Commercial eyedrops clear the eyes by forcing the dilated blood vessels to contract, but this is only a short-term solution, and in the long run does the eyes more damage than good. Better to bath the eyes with a gentle herbal infusion, or simply with half a teaspoon of salt in a glass of purified water.

Red, itchy eyelids often mean an allergy to a cosmetic. If this is a frequent problem stick to hypo-allergenic make-up ranges, or get used to going without eye make-up. You can have your lashes dyed at a beauty salon, and so by-pass the need for mascara.

Falling lashes is the natural result of each lash reaching the end of its growing cycle. A lash only grows for six months before it enters a resting phase when it stops growing and separates from the root. A new hair will form in the follicle, pushing out the old one. The loss may be noticeable when removing mascara, but this is merely the result of the friction dislodging hairs that were about to fall. Never pick off old mascara as it is easy to pull out lashes as well.

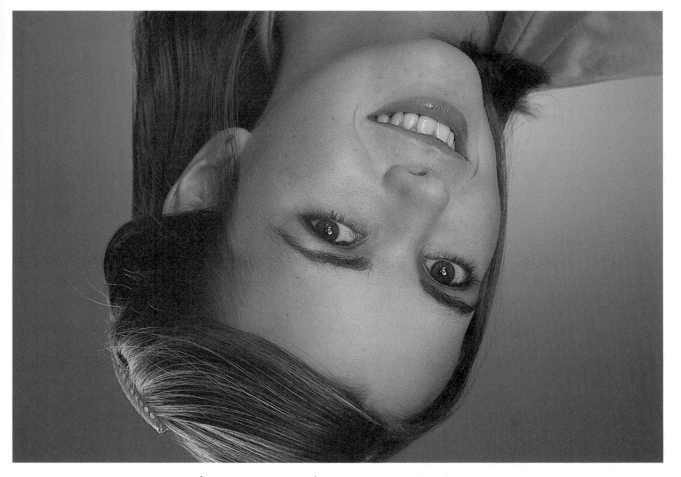

Eye treatments, creams and make-up remover

The eye washes and eyepads featured on this page can be made simply with natural ingredients and do not need a full recipe.

Eyewashes

To clear bloodshot and irritated eyes, cooled decoctions of herbs and flowers are very useful. Boiling the herbs in purified water rather than making an infusion ensures that any bacteria are killed off before use. Use one teaspoon of the herb to a cup of boiling water, and strain them thoroughly through coffee filter paper to remove every tiny particle from the liquid.

The following are all well-known eye herbs:

Eyebright	**Angelica seeds**	**Hyssop**
Cornflowers	**Borage**	**Elderflowers**
Verbena		

To soothe the entire eye area pour the filtered decoctions into an ice-cube tray. When frozen, rub a cube over your eyelids.

Eyepads

Any of the following natural ingredients will help reduce puffiness and really refresh the eyes. Place over the eyes for a short time and completely relax.

Slices of chilled cucumber

Slices of scrubbed and peeled potato

Lukewarm teabags – try camomile or rosehip

Grated apple spread on gauze, placed with gauze side against the eyelids

Witch hazel soaked into cotton wool pads. (Apply a little oil to the eye area first as this may sting).

Any of the herbs used in eyewashes can also be used.

Lanolin and almond oil cream
(1 small pot)
15g (½oz) lanolin
15g (½oz) beeswax
125ml (4fl oz) almond oil
30ml (1½fl oz) rosewater

Melt the lanolin and beeswax in a double boiler (or in a small container in a saucepan of hot water) and add the almond oil. Heat the rosewater separately and remove both pans from the heat. Beat the rosewater into the oil and wax mixture until cool, using a wooden spoon. Pour into screw-top pot. This cream, ideal for dry skin, should be patted around the eyes at night.

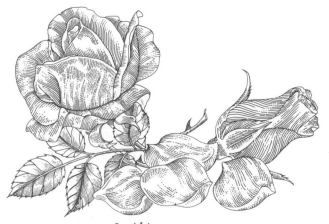

Lecithin eye cream
(1 small pot)
15g (½oz) lanolin
125ml (4fl oz) almond oil
1 teaspoon powdered lecithin
2 teaspoons purified water

Melt the lanolin in a double boiler or in a heat-resistant bowl over hot water and add the almond oil. Remove from the heat and stir in the lecithin until smooth. Add the water and beat together with electric beater or spoon. Pour into screw-top pot. This oily cream contains protein and sinks into the eye area.

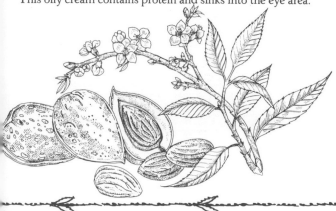

Wheatgerm eye cream
(1 small pot)
15g (½oz) lanolin
½ tablespoon beeswax
½ tablespoon emulsifying wax
3 tablespoons wheatgerm oil
3 tablespoons purified water or rosewater
¼ teaspoon borax
Few drops perfume oil

Melt the lanolin and waxes together in a double boiler or in a heat-resistant bowl over hot water, then add the oil. Heat the water separately and add the borax to the water. Remove pans from heat and beat the water into the wax mixture until cool. Pour into screw-top pot. This rich oil contains vitamin E in the wheatgerm to feed tired and wrinkled skin.

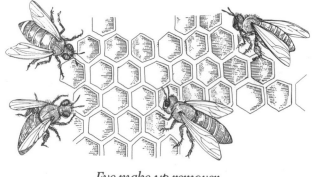

Eye make-up remover
(1 small bottle)
1 tablespoon beeswax
6 tablespoons almond oil
2 tablespoons purified water
1 teaspoon borax

Melt the oil and wax together in a double boiler or in a heat-resistant bowl over hot water, heat the water separately, and stir in the borax. Remove pans from heat and beat the water into the oil and wax mixture, until cool. This light oily cream should remove even stubborn make-up without any added perfume to irritate. You could use two tablespoons of a herbal infusion (see page 20) such as cornflower, but add some benzoin.

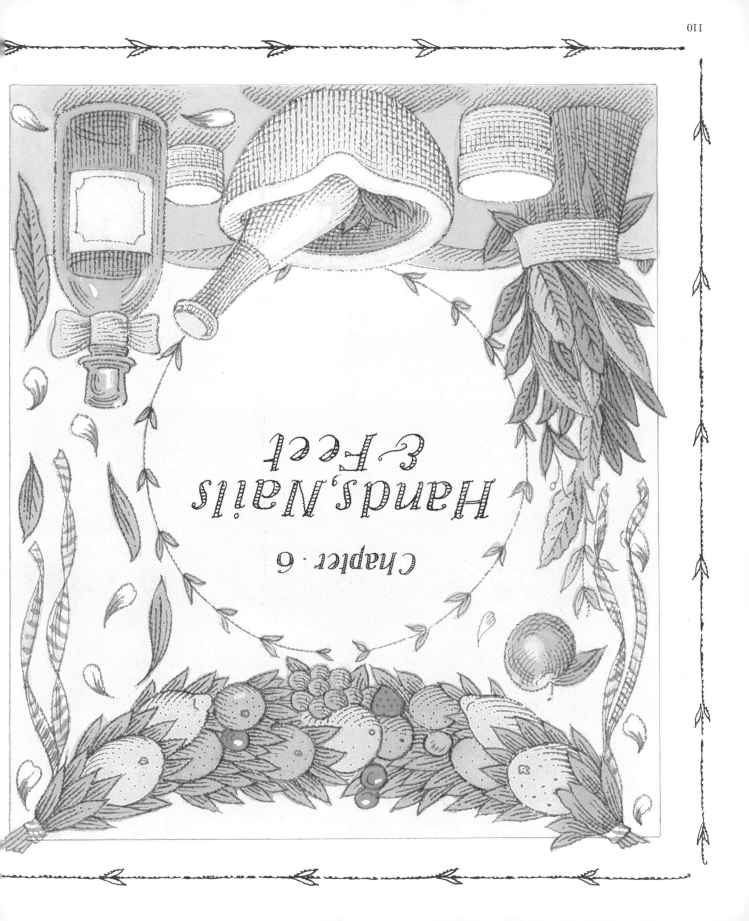

Chapter · 6

Hands, Nails & Feet

The hands, nails and feet are usually the most neglected parts of the body, even though they are also the most hard-working. Your hands and nails are always on show so any neglect is immediately evident, but feet are more easily forgotten as they are hidden away in boots and shoes for the best part of the year. Lavish a little care on your hands and feet as part of your daily beauty routine and the rewards will be immediate. Neglected hands betray their owners immediately. A well-cared for face may possess an ageless beauty – but rough wrinkled hands and broken or chewed nails can make you seem a lot older and spoil your appearance. Rough skin, chipped toenails and callouses can be most unattractive even if the rest of your body is in superb condition. Look after your hands and feet and they will never let you down.

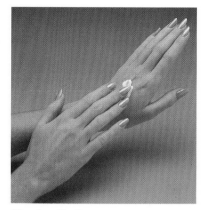

Hands suffer from constant use and exposure to all weather conditions, so they need regular pampering to keep them soft and smooth. Keep jars of your favourite home-made hand cream on your dressing table, in the bathroom and in your desk at work, so that you can moisturize dry hands whenever you find it necessary.

The hands

The so-called ideal feminine hand is slender, white and graceful, with long tapering fingers topped by oval pearly nails. The shape of your hands is hereditary, and short square hands with stubby fingers and brittle nails are unfairly common. But you can do a great deal to improve the overall appearance of your hands with some loving care and attention.

The backs of the hands have little fat and a meagre supply of sebaceous glands – the palms have none at all, although they do have a copious supply of sweat glands which over-act embarrassingly when you feel nervous. The little natural oil that the hands do possess is constantly being stripped away by water, detergents and unsympathetic weather conditions. Consequently they need to be treated with every bit as much care as your face, with constant attention to protection and moisturizing.

Basic hand care

Follow these simple guidelines and you will be doing all that is necessary to keep your hands in peak condition. But care must be constant – forget for a few days and your hands will soon show the neglect.

● **Always protect your** hands from hot water and detergents by wearing gloves when washing up. Try to buy plastic gloves rather than the rubber variety, as your hands will start to sweat after they have been encased in rubber for a while, and this can cause skin problems. Wearing a pair of cotton gloves inside rubber or plastic ones is ideal. Always wear gloves for household cleaning and gardening.

● **Do not wash** your hands with harsh soaps that you would not consider using on your face – the skin on your hands is just as delicate, often more so. Only use mild, naturally perfumed soaps and avoid commercial brands with strong synthetic scents. Dry your hands thoroughly with a soft dry towel after washing and check that the areas under rings and bracelets are dry.

● **Use lashings of** hand cream whenever you feel the need, but particularly

Always wear warm gloves in winter, to protect your hands and in the summer use a sunscreen cream. Hands can become wrinkled and age faster than the face if neglected.

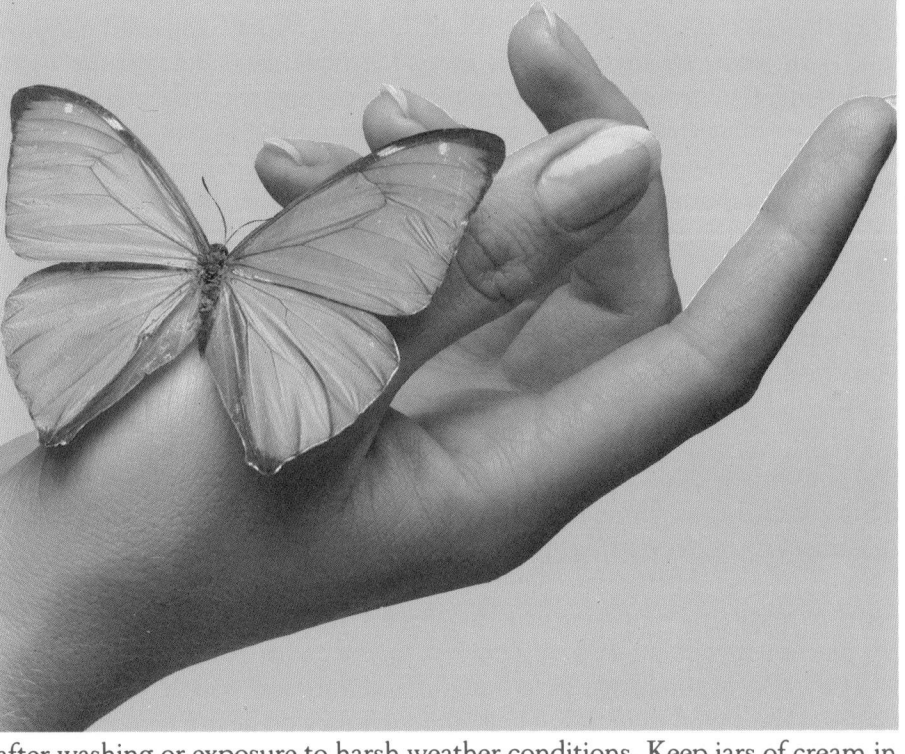

after washing or exposure to harsh weather conditions. Keep jars of cream in the kitchen and bathroom, in the bedroom and at work, so that you can replenish lost oils whenever your hands feel dry.

● **Give your hands** a thorough massage every time you apply hand cream. This will help the cream to be absorbed by the skin, and tone up the circulation. Start at the wrists and work up between the fingers, so encouraging the blood flow to the fingertips. Massage the knuckles and fingertips last.

● **Protect your hands** from the sun by wearing a sunscreen cream. Too much sun not only ages hands by destroying the elasticity of the skin, it also causes brown spots which are giant freckles caused by clusters of melanin. Protect your hands from the cold, too by wearing warm gloves in winter. If you have to go without gloves use a barrier cream (an extra rich moisturizer).

● **Give your hands** an occasional treat with an over-night hand mask. This is an extra thick cream which should be applied lavishly before bed. Protect your sheets by wearing cotton gloves, then wash off the mixture in the morning. Your hands will be beautifully soft and smooth.

● **If your hands** tend to be red because of bad circulation, exercise can help. Try alternately clenching your fists then spreading out your fingers. Then with fingers outstretched, bend each finger into your palm one at a time, keeping the rest of the fingers straight. Camouflage red hands with a little foundation mixed into your hand cream and dust with talcum powder.

The nails

The reason you have fingernails is to protect your sensitive fingertips. The nails fulfil this function very well, but suffer a great deal of damage in the process. We all tend to use our nails as tools for picking, prising and scratching, and nervous types also chew them. Without attention, fingernails can not survive unscathed. They break and split, and the surrounding skin can become sore and inflamed.

Filing the nails into a smooth oval shape is as good for their health as for their appearance. A healthy nail looks smooth and pink, is flexible yet strong and has no white flecks in it. Nails are made from the same keratin cells as those on the surface of the skin, but they are far more tightly compressed together to provide a thicker texture. The live nail cells start growing in the matrix which is about 3mm (⅛in) beneath the visible base of the nail. A tiny patch of live nail can be seen at the white half moon which is called the lunula. If these live cells under the skin are damaged, either by knocks, cuts or general ill health, these will show up later as white flecks and ridges as the cells grow up the visible nail plate. As nails grow fairly slowly – about 1mm (0.4in) a week, ill-health or damage will not show up for several weeks, so it is a myth that your nails reveal your current state of health. It takes about four months for a nail to grow out completely from base to tip, so all you can do for ridges and flecks is to camouflage them with nail varnish.

Basic nail care

Beautiful nails are the reward for care and attention. Follow these guidelines and you will achieve fingertips that are a beauty asset rather than a flaw.
- **Never cut or** use nail varnish remover on your cuticles – the area of skin that grows round the base of the nail to protect the vulnerable base cells beneath. If cuticles are growing up too far, push them back gently with a towel every time you dry your hands, or use a cotton bud dipped in oil. Never pick at your cuticles while the skin is dry as this can result in 'hangnails' (nails with torn skin) and sore flaking skin.
- **Keep your nails** fairly short, as long ones are very likely to break and can look unattractive. To achieve the right shape, file the nails with a long emery board, not a metal file which can split the nails. Start filing with the rough side of the emery board, using long strokes from side to centre. Aim for an oval shape, then use the smoother side of the board to finish off.
- **Keep the nails clean**, but never poke sharp instruments underneath the free edge to remove dirt. Soak the fingertips in a mild soapy solution, and scrub with a soft nail brush.
- **Rub hand cream** into your nails each time you apply it to your hands. Nails dry out just like skin when neglected.
- **Buff your nails** into a shine with a chamois buffer. This also helps to stimulate the circulation at the fingertips, so feeding the growing nails.

Below and bottom: Do not grow your nails too long as they split and can break easily. Aim for a smooth oval shape. Regular manicures help strong nails to grow. Never clean the nails by poking sharp instruments under the free edge – scrub them with warm soapy water and a soft nail brush.

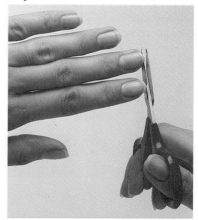

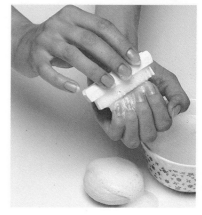

Hand creams, conditioning treatments and nail strengtheners

Rosewater and glycerine hand lotion
(1 small bottle)
4 tablespoons glycerine
6 tablespoons rosewater

Mix the two ingredients together and bottle. To make a thicker cream, add 2 tablespoons of cornflour. You can also add a ½ teaspoon of cider vinegar and a ½ teaspoon of honey – this will help to make the cream more nourishing.

Coconut oil hand cream
(1 small bottle)
1 tablespoons beeswax
2 tablespoons almond oil
1 tablespoon coconut oil
2 tablespoons glycerine

Melt the wax and oils together in a double boiler or in a heat-resistant bowl over hot water. Take off the heat and add the glycerine very slowly until a creamy consistency is produced. Pour into a small bottle. This rich oily cream is absorbed quickly into the hands leaving them feeling smooth and soft.

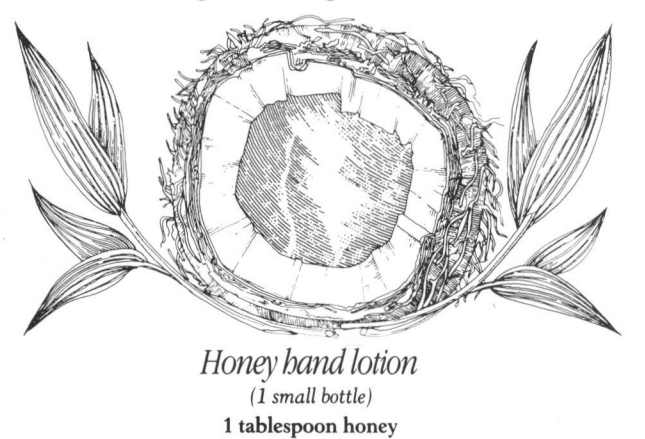

Honey hand lotion
(1 small bottle)
1 tablespoon honey
1 teaspoon emulsifying wax
1 tablespoon almond oil
4 tablespoons rosewater
½ tablespoon cider vinegar

Warm the honey in a double boiler or in a heat-resistant bowl over hot water, and then add the almond oil and wax. Remove the mixture from the heat and slowly add rosewater and vinegar, beating together well, and bottle. This lotion is particularly good for very dry hands.

Almond hand lotion
(1 small bottle)
60g (2oz) ground almonds
6 tablespoons rosewater
½ teaspoon grated soap
1 teaspoon glycerine

Pound the almonds in half the rosewater until you get a milky paste, then strain through muslin. Warm the soap with the glycerine and the remainder of rosewater in a double boiler or in a heat-resistant bowl over hot water, add to the almond milk. Strain the mixture through muslin and bottle. This cream is an excellent remedy for red roughened hands.

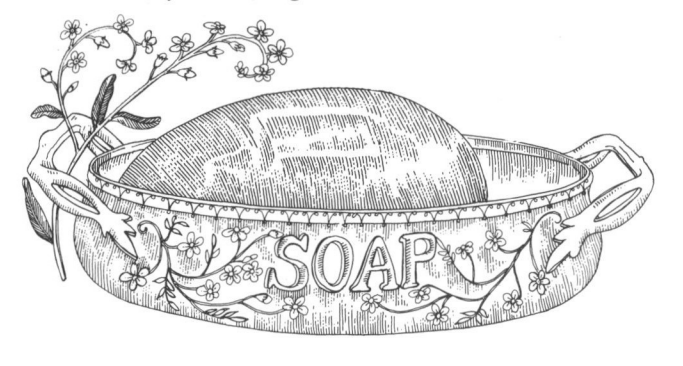

Lanolin hand cream
(1 small bottle)
25g (1oz) lanolin
2 tablespoons almond oil
2 tablespoons glycerine
Few drops of geranium oil

Melt the lanolin in a double boiler or in heat-resistant bowl over hot water, and add the almond oil and glycerine. Remove from the heat and beat well. When cool, add the perfume oil.

Barrier cream (to protect working hands)
(3 applications)
2 egg yolks
2 teaspoons kaolin or fullers' earth
1 teaspoon almond oil

Mix all the ingredients together until they form a paste. Keep the paste chilled in the fridge all the time. Apply liberally to the backs of the hands only.

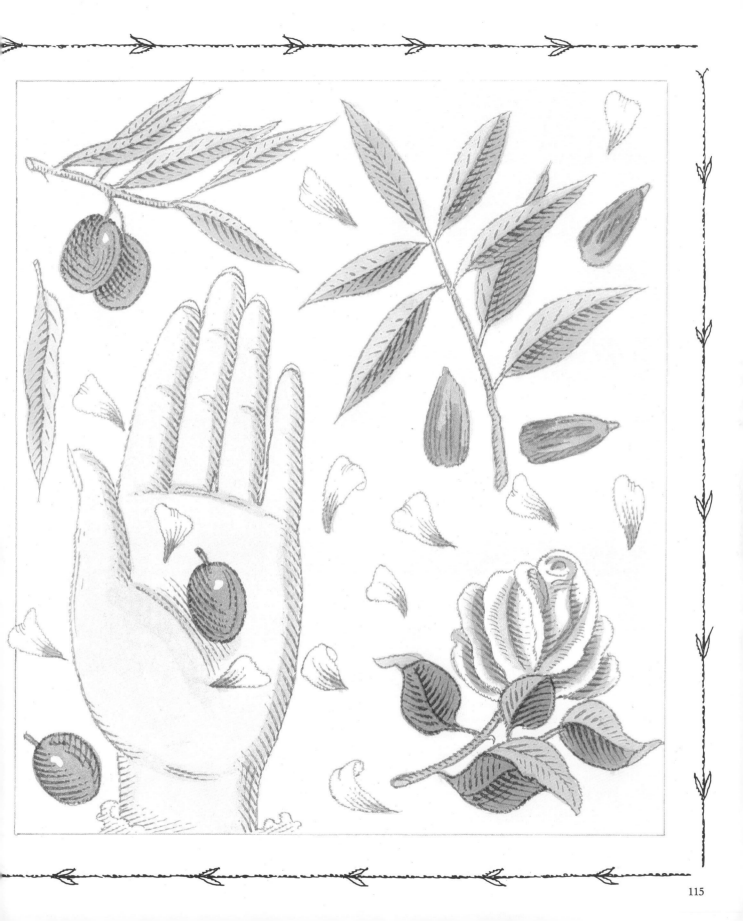

Almond night cream
(1 small bottle)
2 teaspoons ground almonds
4 teaspoons almond oil
1 teaspoon rosewater
1 egg yolk

Beat the egg yolk into the ground almonds, then add the almond oil and water, beating hard, and bottle. You can smooth this thick cream over the hands last thing at night and cover with cotton gloves. Rinse the cream off thoroughly in the morning for smooth, softer hands.

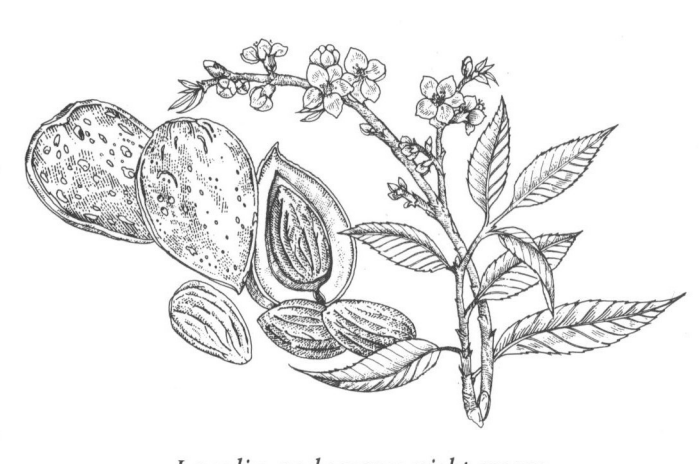

Lanolin and sesame night cream
(2 applications)
25g (1oz) lanolin
1 tablespoon sesame oil

Melt the oils together in a double boiler or in a heat-resistant bowl over hot water. Remove from heat and beat firmly until a cream is formed. Pour into wide-topped bottle. When cool rub into the hands and cover them with cotton gloves. Rinse off in the morning.

Honey night oil
(2 applications)
1 teaspoon honey
1 tablespoon almond oil
1 tablespoon olive oil
½ tablespoon glycerine

Warm the honey until it runs and then add both the oils and glycerine. Beat them well together and pour into wide-lipped bottle. When cool massage this rich oil well into your hands and put on cotton gloves. Rinse off the oil thoroughly in the morning to leave soft hands.

Lemon and iodine nail lotion
(1 application)
2 teaspoons lemon juice
2 teaspoons iodine solution

Mix ingredients together and paint onto the nails at night. This lotion both strengthens and whitens the nails.

Honey and avocado nail cream
(1 application)
1 teaspoon honey
1 teaspoon avocado oil
1 egg yolk
½ teaspoon kaolin

Mix all ingredients together to make a nourishing paste and rub into the nails. Leave for half an hour and rinse off.

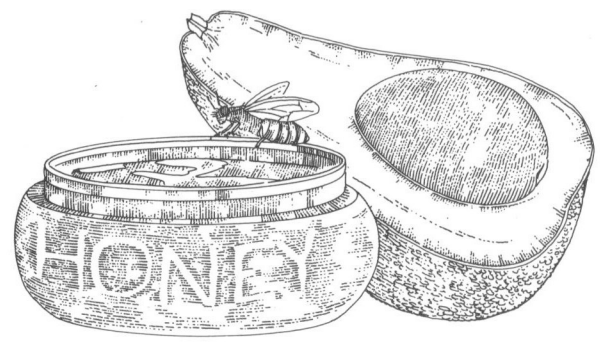

Lecithin and olive oil nail cream
(1 application)
2 teaspoons olive oil
2 teaspoons lecithin powder

Mix to form a smooth paste and rub into nails. Leave for half an hour and rinse off. This paste is particularly good to use for brittle nails.

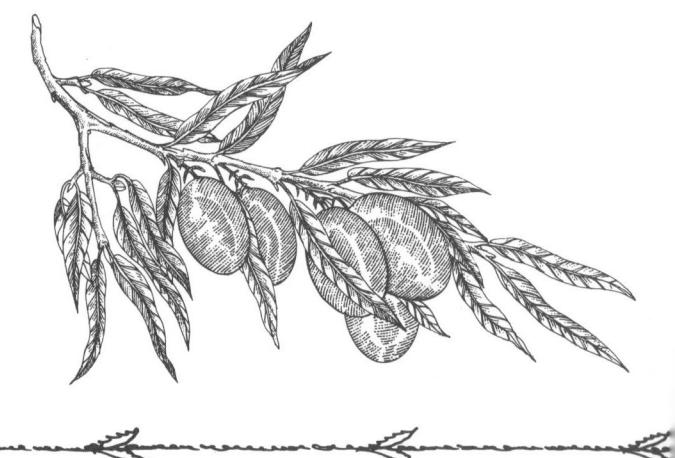

The feet

Neglect your feet and you will soon begin to suffer with blisters, corns and hard skin. Most people are born with perfect feet, but they often grow deformed and ugly from misuse. Feet were not meant to be crammed into pointed shoes, and their natural arches are not equipped to stand the constant strain of high heels. The soles of the feet perspire liberally, and infections can result from wearing nylon hosiery and plastic shoes. Few women are willing to wear 'sensible' footwear all the time, so the next best action is to pamper your feet regularly to restore them to perfect health.

Even the most sensibly shod can develop tired aching feet and swollen ankles from long hours of standing or walking. Body fluids tend to accumulate around the ankles at the end of the day, leading to puffiness.

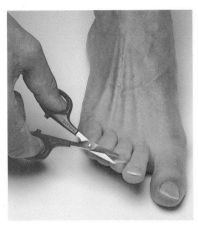

Toenails should be kept short, and clipped straight across with nail scissors or clippers. They should not be shaped at the sides as this can cause painful, ingrowing toenails.

Basic foot care

● **Choose shoes** with low heels for everyday wear. The maximum height should be 6cm (2½in) for day wear, and they should be exchanged for flat shoes at least once a day to avoid straining the feet, legs and back.

● **Keep the feet** as clean as possible. Wash them every day in warm soapy water, and rub away any rough skin with a pumice stone.

● **Cut your toenails** regularly. Trim them straight across – do not try to shape the sides as this can lead to painful ingrowing toenails.

● **Rest aching feet** and swollen ankles by lying down with feet raised a few millimetres above your body. Then give them a reviving massage by pressing all over the soles with your thumbs in a circular movement.

● **Best of all**, treat your feet to a herbal foot balm in warm water. It will leave your feet feeling pampered and refreshed.

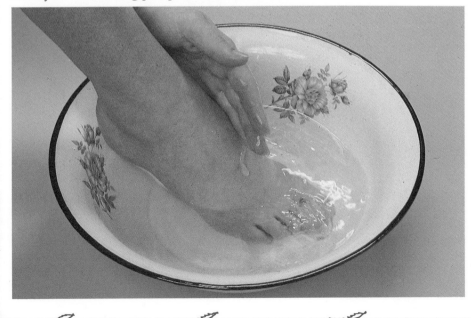

Foot balms

Herbal foot bath (For aching feet)
(1 application)
1 tablespoon each of rosemary, camomile, peppermint, thyme and yarrow
1 tablespoon washing soda

Make an infusion of all the above ingredients in a pint of boiling, purified water. Strain through a sieve and add to a foot bath of warm water, then add the washing soda. Relax feet in the foot bath and let this soothing balm do its work. Pat feet dry and apply a hand lotion, or dust with talcum powder.

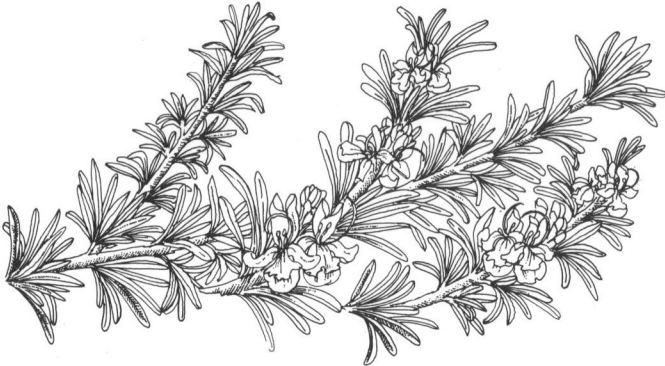

Lavender foot balm
(1 application)
1-2 tablespoons dried lavender flowers
1 teaspoon lavender oil

Fill a bowl with warm water and add the lavender and the lavender oil. This flower is particularly refreshing to aching feet.

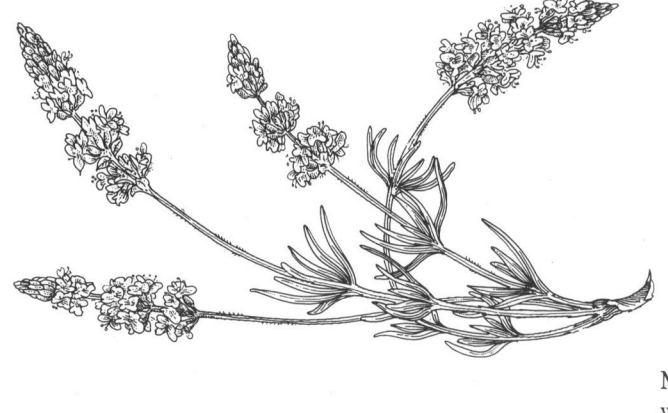

Epsom salts foot soak
(1 application)
1 tablespoon epsom salts
1 tablespoon borax

Mix together in a bowl of hot water and soak tired feet.

Nettle and vinegar foot balm
(1 application)
1 tablespoon nettles
1 tablespoon cider vinegar

Make an infusion with the nettles and add to a bowl of hot water, then add the cider vinegar.

Mustard foot bath
(1 application)
1 teaspoon mustard powder

Add the mustard powder to a bowl of hot water. This foot bath is very stimulating for tired or cold feet as it helps the circulation.

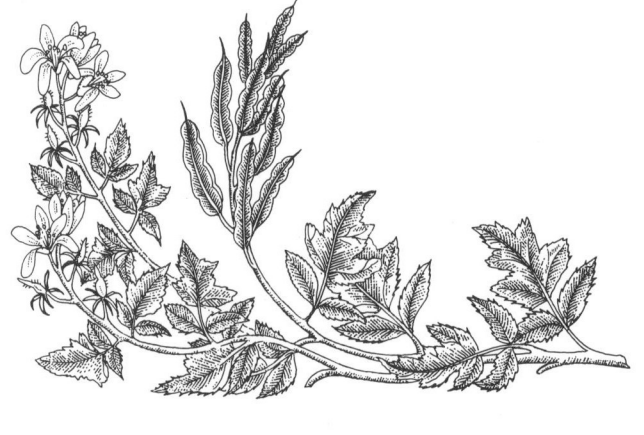

Foot massage oil
(1 application)
3 tablespoons olive, almond or sesame oil
6 drops of clove oil

Mix the oils together and massage into the feet, working hard with the thumbs to relieve aches and pains.

Bibliography

Culpeper, Culpeper's Complete Herbal, W, Foulsham & Co., London
Dincin Buchman D., An ABC Of Natural Beauty
Eagle R., Herbs, Useful Plants, BBC publications 1981
Genders R., Growing Herbs, Hodder and Stoughton 1980
Grieve M.A., Modern Herbal Penguin Books, 1976
Griggs B., Green Pharmacy A History Of Herbal Medicine, Jill Norman & Hobhouse 1981
Grigson G., The Englishman's Flora, Paladin Books 1975
Growing Herbs, The Herb Society 1977
Keble M.W., The Concise British Flora In Colour, Sphere Books 1972
Kresanek J., Plants That Heal, Galley Press 1982
Law D., The Concise Herbal Encyclopedia, John Bartholomew 1982
Maxwell-Hudson C., The Natural Beauty Book, Macdonald 1976
Meredith B., Natural Health and Beauty, Penguin Books 1981
Murray D. Scientific Skincare, Arlington Books 1983
Palaiseul J., Grandmother's Secrets, Penguin 1976
Readers Digest Encyclopedia of Garden Plants And Flowers, The Readers Digest Association 1978

Useful Addresses

The Herb Society
77 Great Peter Street
London
SW1
telephone: 01-222-3634
(For information)

Baldwins
173 Walworth Road
London
SE17
telephone: 01-703-5550
(stocks herbs, oils etc)

Culpeper Ltd
Hadstock Road
Linton
Cambridge
CB1 6NJ
telephone: Cambridge 891196
(Herbalists) Culpeper has branches around the country, and a mail order service.

John Bell & Croydon
52 Wigmore Street
London
W1H 0AU
telephone: 01-935-5555
(A wide selection of pharmaceuticals and oils)

Gerard House
736b Christchurch Road
Boscombe
Bournemouth
BH7 6Z
telephone: Bournemouth 35352
(Mail order herbs and essential oils)

Picture credits
Aromatherapy Handbook/Century: 44
Walter Bauer: 24
Tom Belshaw: 100, 102
Steve Bicknell: 20, 23, 66, 95, 101
Steve Bielschowsky: 65, 69
Tony Boase: 92
Bodleian Library: 8
Camera Press: 13(t)
Anthony Denney: 14(r)
Alan Duns: Endpapers, 1, 4/5, 73(1), 84
Ray Duns: 2/3, 38
Geoffrey Frosh: 71
John Garrett: 46
Hank Kemme: 58
David Levin: 19(t,b)
Di Lewis: 62(b)
Sandra Lousada: 52
Maison de Marie Claire/Godeaut: 75
Mansell Collection: 7, 28, 32(t), 39, 45(b)
Brian Nash: 117(b)
Roger Phillips: 22
Colin Ramsey: 67
Royal Horticultural Society: 26, 31, 35
Kim Sayer: 63, 94, 107
Harry Smith: 16
Tony Stone Associates: 70
Graham Strong: 62(t)
Sungravure: 50
Ron Sutherland: 61
Pamela Toler: 13(b), 14(1)
Jerry Tubby: 12
Michael Wickham: 11(t,b)
Paul Winsor: 112, 113, 117(t)

Illustrations
Ian Beck: 6, 10, 15, 18, 21, 54, 59, 88, 93, 110, 115
Ian Garrard: 25
Vana Haggerty: 9, 17, 27, 29, 30, 32(b), 33, 34, 36, 40-43, 45(t), 47-49, 51, 53, 60, 64, 72, 73(r), 83, 85-87, 96-99, 103, 104, 109, 114, 116, 118, 119
Frank Kennard: 89
Aziz Khan: 56

Index

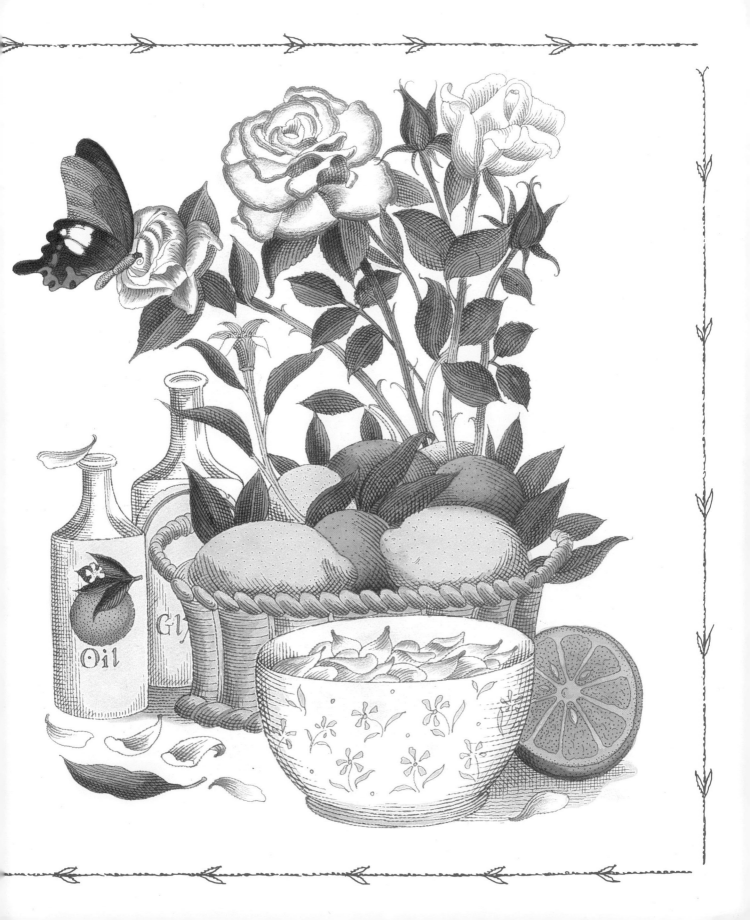

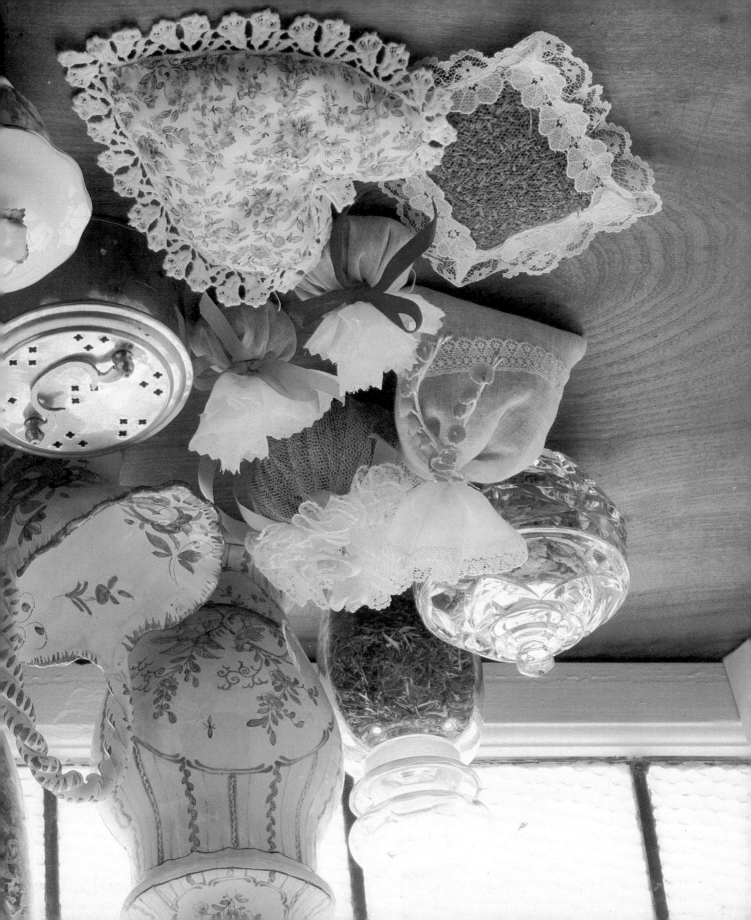